Latinos in NURSING

Invisible No More: The Legacy and Honor of Latino Nurses

Tina Loarte-Rodríguez

This book is a compilation of stories from numerous people who have each contributed a chapter and is designed to provide inspiration to our readers.

It is sold with the understanding that the publisher and the individual authors are not engaged in the rendering of psychological, legal, accounting, or other professional advice. The content and views in each chapter are the sole expression and opinion of its author and not necessarily the views of Transformative Leadership Revolution, LLC.

For more information visit:
Latinas in Nursing |www.latinasinnursing.org

Cover Design by Brian Ochoa Design
www.brianochoadesign.com

Layout by Tina Loarte-Rodríguez

Printed in the United States of America

ISBN: ISBN: 978-1-967769-00-1
Library of Congress Control Number: 2025908927

TLR
TRANSFORMATIVE LEADERSHIP REVOLUTION, LLC

For my *manitos*—

The ones who were told nursing wasn't for them,
Who walked into rooms where they weren't expected,
And stayed—because our communities needed them to.

To the brothers who care quietly,
Lead boldly,
And carry generations of strength in their hearts and hands.
This is for you.

For your legacy, your sacrifice, your brilliance.
May these pages honor your journey,
And remind the world that you've always been here.

Con orgullo y respeto, siempre.

TABLE OF CONTENTS

Acknowledgements

With deep gratitude and immense pride, I acknowledge the many hearts and hands that helped bring this inaugural *Latinos in Nursing* book to life.

To the first Latino male nurses who paved the way—often in silence and in the shadows—thank you for being the roots of a legacy we are only now beginning to name aloud. One of the earliest known Latino male nurses in U.S. history, Dr Hector Hugo Gonzalez, was the first registered nurse to earn his PhD, transforming nursing education and champioing diversity thoughout the profession.

To today's leaders like Dr. Elias Provencio-Vasquez and Dr. Julian L. Gallegos—your work, scholarship, and advocacy have opened doors for a generation of Latino nurses who now know they belong in the boardroom, the classroom, and the research lab. Your visibility matters. Your voices matter. Your presence in this profession is powerful beyond measure.

To the contributors of this inaugural anthology—you are the soul of this book. Thank you for your vulnerability, your stories, your brilliance, and your strength. Your words carry weight. They build bridges. They challenge narratives and create space where space has long been denied. You are not just part of the story—you are reshaping the future of nursing.

To my family—thank you for being my grounding force and my greatest source of joy. Your patience, encouragement, and unconditional love fuel my purpose and sustain me when the work feels heavy. This project, like so much of what I do, is rooted in the values you instilled in me and nurture: faith, service, justice, and *comunidad*.

To the supporters, advisors, and believers who have stood beside me through the launch and growth of this series—thank you. You've helped transform an idea into a movement. Your belief in the importance of telling our stories has made this moment possible.

This book marks the beginning of a revolution in how we see and celebrate Latino nurses. It is the first volume in a series that will continue to elevate our voices, affirm our existence, and reclaim our place in the profession.

To every Latino nurse reading this—past, present, and future—you are seen, you are valued, and you belong.

Con poder y con corazón,
Dra. Tina

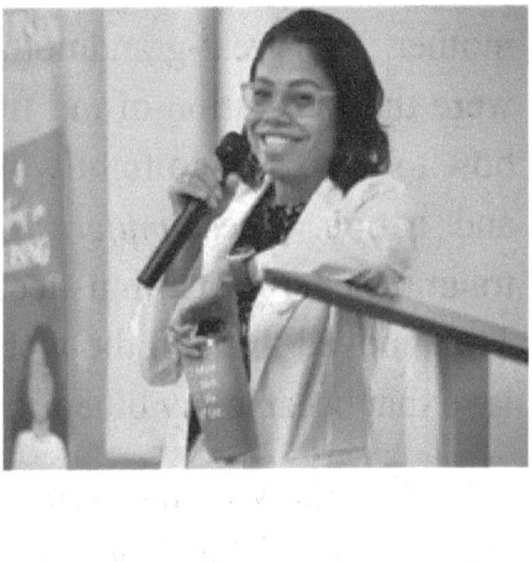

Foreword

I am the first in my family to earn a PhD in nursing. The first Chicano Nursing Theorist. The first Chicano male faculty at Purdue University. And the first Chicano appointed to the Indiana State Board of Nursing and the American Nurse Credentialing Center Board of Directors.

But I did not walk this path alone.

My story begins in the rural northern regions of New Mexico, where my roots run deep through the *sangre* of both Spanish and Native American ancestors. These lands are rugged, sacred, and soaked in culture and tradition. It is here, among the adobe homes and mountains that touch the sky, that my people endured hardship, held on to their faith, and passed down a powerful mix of heritage that shaped who I am today.

After my father passed away when I was just three years old, I was raised by a lineage of strong, unshakable Latina women, my mother, my great-grandmother, and my great-great aunt. They were the foundation of my life. They taught me how to love and how to lead, how to fight with heart, and how to heal with words and action. These *mujeres* carried the weight of generational trauma, poverty, and injustice, but never allowed it to define them. They moved through the world with a quiet strength and a fierce love that became my blueprint.

When my mother remarried, my stepfather became another crucial part of that story. A man who taught me the meaning of integrity, discipline, and compassion in a different way. Through his love and guidance, I became a man who was not afraid to break expectations, especially in a culture where *machismo* often dictates who you can and cannot be.

In communities like mine, nursing was not traditionally seen as a career for men, let alone Chicano men. The pressures to conform to hypermasculine roles were real. But I pushed through them. Not just for myself, but for every young Latino boy who needed to see that there is strength in compassion, that healing is a form of leadership, and that *we* belong in this profession too.

This book, *Latinos in Nursing*, is more than a celebration. It's a declaration. It says: **We are here. We belong. And we are leading.**

Latinos now make up nearly 20% of the U.S. population, yet less than 8% of the nursing workforce reflects that reality. This isn't just a discrepancy; it's a moral failure. Our absence in healthcare doesn't just mean fewer jobs or titles, it means our communities are underserved, our patients are misunderstood, and lives are lost because cultural gaps are left unfilled.

Representation in healthcare matters. *We* matter.

As Latino nurses, we bring more than clinical knowledge, we bring our culture, our language, and our lived experience. We are the trusted face for patients who feel forgotten. We are the voice for the voiceless, the translator in times of confusion, and the advocate in rooms where decisions are made. We don't just heal bodies, we heal systems.

And yet, the systems we work within are not always welcoming.

We are navigating a political and professional climate that is increasingly hostile to diversity, equity, and inclusion. Anti-DEI rhetoric has grown louder, often undermining the very principles of fairness and representation that our communities depend on. At the same time, healthcare inequities continue to hit our people the hardest. We see it in the emergency rooms, the clinics, and the COVID statistics that disproportionately affected Latino families.

But we are not standing still. *We are the response to inequity.*

Latino nurses are not just caregivers, we are also leaders, educators, researchers, and community builders. We are dismantling barriers from within. We are asking hard questions. We are mentoring the next generation so that the "firsts" become many and eventually become the norm.

Still, the barriers are real. From the moment we consider nursing as a career, we face systemic hurdles in recruitment, admission, retention, and advancement. There are too few of us at the top, in leadership roles, in academia, in research, and on regulatory boards. That's why visibility and mentorship are not just important, they are **urgently necessary**.

That's why this book matters.

Latinos in Nursing isn't just a collection of stories, it's a movement. It's a tool for change. It's a mirror and a map. It reflects where we've been and points to where we need to go. You will read stories from pioneers and trailblazers. You'll see yourself in their triumphs, their pain, and their dreams. You'll walk away knowing that *you are not alone* and that you are part of something much bigger than yourself.

Representation in nursing doesn't just improve outcomes. It shifts culture. It redefines excellence. It reminds the world that excellence does not have one face, one accent, or one zip code. It lives in our italize barrio, our rural communities, our immigrant households, and in every student who dares to dream beyond what they were told they could be.

To the Latino student wondering if they belong in nursing school, you do.

To the new graduate navigating the system for the first time, keep going.

To the seasoned nurse ready to lead, step forward.

To every Chicano, Chicana, and Latinx nurse reading this book, you are not the "only one." And even if you are today, you won't be tomorrow. Because we're changing that. Together.

As the first Chicano Nursing Theorist, I created a framework that centers our experiences and cultural values on men's health. As the first Chicano appointed to the Indiana State Board of Nursing and American Nurse Credentialing Center Board of Directors, I carry the responsibility of opening doors and challenging systems that were not built for us. And as the first Chicano male faculty at Purdue, I mentor, teach, and lead not just for myself, but for every student watching me break the mold.

I say this not out of pride, but out of purpose. These "firsts" only matter if they are followed by many more. And that is the mission of this book, to inspire, equip, and ignite the next generation of Latino nurses.

Our presence in this profession is not an accident. It is the result of generations of sacrifice. Of *abuelos* who prayed, mothers and fathers who worked double shifts, and communities who believed in us before we believed in ourselves. We stand on their shoulders, and we now have a duty to build even stronger foundations for those who come next.

To every reader of this book: Let these stories be your fire. Let them give you hope. Let them remind you that your heritage is not a barrier, it is your strength.

Be proud. Be bold. Be the voice that your community needs.

We are not guests in nursing. We are its future.

Julian L. Gallegos, PhD, MBA, APRN, FNPBC, CNL, CMHE, FAUNA

Assistant Professor, Assistant Head of Graduate Programs
Purdue University – West Lafayette

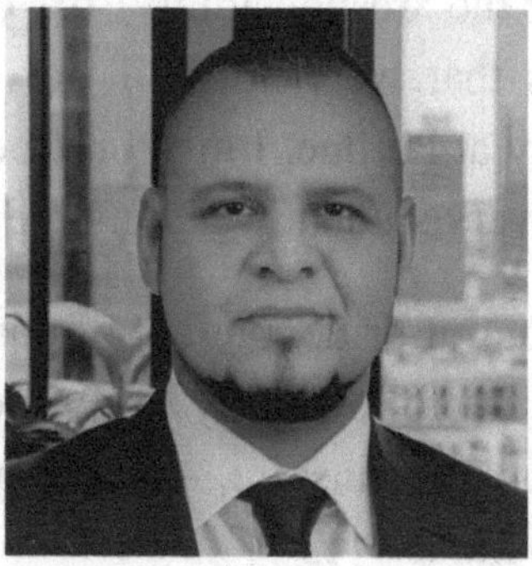

Introduction

Reclaiming Our Place in Nursing
The Rise of Latinos in the Profession

Nursing is often described as a calling—a profession built on compassion, healing, and human connection. But beneath its noble surface lies a complex history shaped by exclusion, colonization, and structural inequities. The image of the nurse as a white woman in crisp scrubs has been carefully crafted over time. It's familiar, iconic—and incomplete.

Latinos—men and women—have always been caretakers. From the *curanderos* of Mesoamerica to community caregivers rooted in traditions passed down for generations, we have healed bodies, tended to spirits, and supported families long before professional nursing was formalized. Yet, our contributions have been undervalued, our presence underrepresented, and our voices, until now, largely unheard.

This anthology is more than a collection of stories—it's a declaration. A reclamation. A reminder that Latinos are not new to nursing—we are foundational to it. And now, we are rising.

Let's break a myth: nursing was not always a "women's profession." In ancient societies, including Greece and Rome, men were primary caregivers. In medieval Europe, monastic communities—largely male—provided nursing care to the poor and sick. Even during the U.S. Civil War, men served as frontline nurses, tending to the wounded in makeshift hospitals and battlefields.

But over time, particularly in the post-Florence Nightingale era, the narrative shifted. As white women began entering the workforce in socially sanctioned roles, nursing became feminized and professionalized in their image. This shift opened doors for one group but closed them for others. Male nurses were sidelined, and men of color—Latino men included—were all but erased from the profession's visual and institutional identity.

Nursing as a profession did not evolve in a vacuum—it was colonized. While caregiving traditions exist across every culture, the Western model of nursing was systematized within a white, Eurocentric framework. What counted as "real" knowledge was narrowly defined. Indigenous healing practices were dismissed. Language, culture, and tradition were seen as liabilities instead of strengths.

Latino communities have always had their own ways of healing—through herbs, prayer, touch, spirit, and family. These practices were often labeled unscientific or primitive by the institutions that dominated healthcare, and the people who carried this wisdom were excluded from formal spaces of training and practice. As nursing developed into a profession, it became not only gendered but racialized. By the early 20th century, the modern nurse was defined by whiteness, modesty, and obedience—qualities deemed incompatible with the presence of Black, Indigenous, and Latino nurses.

The result? A system that claimed to care for all but was built for only a few.

As of July 1, 2023, Latinos comprise 19.5% of the U.S. population, numbering approximately 65.2 million individuals (U.S. Census Bureau, 2024). Despite this significant presence, Latinos are markedly underrepresented in the nursing profession.

Recent data indicates that only about 7% of registered nurses in the U.S. identify as Hispanic or Latino (American Association of Colleges of Nursing, 2024). The numbers become even more sobering when we look at Latino men. While men overall make up about 11% of nurses, Latino men represent just a sliver of that—less than 2% of the nursing workforce (Gallegos, 2023).

Let's be clear: this is not a pipeline problem—it's a systems problem. Latino men are not "missing" from nursing. They have been systematically excluded, underserved, and underestimated.

Latino men encounter numerous obstacles in pursuing and advancing within nursing. Cultural stigma around gender roles in the profession persists. Many Latino boys grow up without ever seeing a man in scrubs as a role model. First-generation students often face financial barriers, limited access to culturally affirming education, and lack of mentorship. Even once in the profession, Latino men may be tokenized, overlooked for leadership, or discouraged from pursuing academic advancement. Bias and exclusion are not just challenges to overcome; they are structural realities that demand systemic change.

Representation matters. It is not just about appearance; it impacts health outcomes. Patients have better experiences and results when cared for by providers who understand their culture and speak their language. For Latino communities facing persistent disparities, this can mean the difference between trust and fear, access and alienation, prevention and crisis.

The stories in this anthology challenge stereotypes and expose truth. They are not just stories of survival or success—they are stories of power, purpose, and presence. They are evidence that Latino nurses, especially men, do not lack talent or commitment. What they lack is access, opportunity, and institutional support.

We must do more than celebrate diversity—we must create systems that foster equity. Academic institutions, healthcare systems, and professional organizations must examine their structures and ask hard questions. Who is being recruited, and who is being left out? Who is leading, and who is being overlooked? Who is being mentored, and who is being sponsored?

Mentorship is essential, but sponsorship is transformative. It means using one's power and privilege to open doors, elevate voices, and create real pathways for Latino nurses to thrive. This includes nominating Latino nurses for leadership roles, including them in decisionmaking spaces, and ensuring their work is visible and valued.

If you are a nurse leader, educator, policymaker, or ally, this is your invitation. Do not just support Latino nurses in word—do it in action. Challenge the status quo. Use your influence. Build the profession we all deserve.

Latino men in nursing are not anomalies. You are not unicorns. You are essential.

This anthology is a mirror and a megaphone. It reflects the brilliance of Latino nurses and amplifies the urgent call for change. Let it move you to think, to feel, and most importantly, to act.

Because the future of nursing is Latino.

And that future begins now—with you.

Tina Loarte-Rodríguez, DNP, RN, CPPS, CPHRM

References

• American Association of Colleges of Nursing. (2024, April). *Nursing Workforce Fact Sheet.* https://www.aacnnursing.org/news-data/fact-sheets/nursing-workforce-fact-sheet

• Gallegos, J. L. (2023). *The underrepresentation of Hispanic male nurses and its implications.* LinkedIn. https://www.linkedin.com/pulse/underrepresentation-hispanic-male-nurses-its-mens-julian

• U.S. Census Bureau. (2024, June 20). *Hispanic Population in the United States: 2023.* U.S. Department of Commerce. https://www.census.gov/data/tables/2023/demo/hispanic-origin/2023-cps.html

Reader Discretion & Support Resources

Content Notice

This anthology contains personal stories that discuss traumatic experiences, including rape, sexual abuse, and suicidal ideation. These narratives are shared with courage and vulnerability to honor the truth and resilience of our contributors.

If you have experienced abuse or are struggling with thoughts of suicide, you are not alone—and help is available. Please consider reaching out to a mental health professional, a trusted support person, or one of the resources below:

National Sexual Assault Hotline: 1-800-656-HOPE (4673) or rainn.org

988 Suicide & Crisis Lifeline: Dial or text **988** or visit 988lifeline.org

You deserve healing. You deserve support.

LATINOS IN NURSING

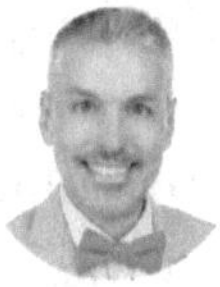

Breaking Barriers, Building Futures: A Piece of Paper, a Promise, and the Journey of a Latino Nurse

RICK GARCÍA

"As we continue to climb, we must reach back and lift those coming behind us—because true success is not just about rising, but about rising together. Come with me!"

"Mientras seguimos ascendiendo, debemos extender la mano y levantar a quienes vienen detrás de nosotros—porque el verdadero éxito no se trata solo de subir, sino de subir juntos. ¡Ven conmigo!"

Current Position

I am the Chief Executive Officer of the Organization for Associate Degree Nursing (OADN) and the OADN Foundation.

What I Love About Nursing

What I love about nursing is the privilege of being present during the most vulnerable moments in someone's life. It's a profession grounded in compassion, science, and service. Nursing allows me to heal, teach, advocate, and lead—all while continuously learning and giving back to the community that shaped me.

Reaching Back: My Journey as a Latino Nurse

I never thought I'd become a nurse. Growing up in a tight-knit Hispanic family, our world was filled with strong traditions, deep-rooted values, and an unshakable sense of community. But nursing? That wasn't something I saw many Latino men doing. It just wasn't on the radar. Yet when I look back now, every moment, every experience—even the ones I didn't understand at the time—was preparing me for this path.

The real foundation, though, started at home. My parents—humble, hardworking, and deeply principled—poured everything into raising me as their firstborn. For nine years, I was their only child. Then came my sister, the result of some persistent encouragement from my maternal grandmother, who insisted it was time for another baby. Eventually, my mother caved—and our family grew.

Even with the challenges they faced, my parents always carried a deep sense of purpose and pride. They knew the value of hard work, but they also knew that to get ahead in this world—especially as a Latino family—we needed more than grit. We needed credentials. My mother had a mantra, one she repeated so often it became part of my internal script: *You can do whatever you want—as long as you earn a piece of paper that tells the world you went to college.*

That piece of paper wasn't just about education. It represented dignity. Credibility. A signal to the world that we were capable, prepared, and deserving of opportunity. That message—spoken over kitchen tables, in the car on the way to school, or as I headed out the door for yet another practice or meeting—grounded me. It shaped how I saw myself and formed my vision of what was possible.

Discovering a Path in High School

In high school, those early seeds began to take root. We were teenagers, but in Mrs. Meyer's class, we were already becoming something more. She had this way of teaching that went beyond textbooks. I still remember the cream of tartar. She had us using it on dental molds—a mirror and an explorer, tiny tools in hand, focused, steady. We weren't just playing around. We were testing our manual dexterity and, in doing so, exploring if we had what it took to pursue something like dental hygiene. That one lesson lit a spark for some of my classmates. For me, it opened a door.

Medical terminology was next. Word by word, we were learning the language of healthcare. It wasn't just about passing a quiz. It was about learning how to communicate in a system we hoped to be part of. It gave us a glimpse of who we could become.

Every December, while other classes were winding down, we were gearing up. Mrs. Meyer had us certified in CPR before we ever left for winter break. At the time, I didn't fully grasp what that meant. Now I see it clearly—we were being prepared, not just academically, but practically, for real responsibility.

She believed in us so deeply that when the opportunity came to join HOSA—the Health Occupations Students of America—she encouraged me to try something totally unexpected: parliamentary procedure. I had no idea what that even was. But I joined the debate team, and with her support, we won regionally, then at the state level, and eventually placed nationally. That experience taught me how to speak up, how to lead, and how to collaborate—all skills that would serve me well beyond the competition floor.

CHOE: The Bridge Between School and Career

And then there was CHOE—Cooperative Health Occupation Education. It was a state-wide, science-based program designed for high school students who were serious about pursuing a career in healthcare. At the time, it felt like a big deal—and looking back, it absolutely was.

CHOE gave us more than just classroom knowledge. It gave us the chance to work, earn, and learn—all while still in high school. That was powerful. I was able to spend part of my school day out in the real world, gaining hands-on experience in healthcare settings, earning a paycheck, and learning how to show up as a professional. We weren't just students anymore—we were contributors, observers, and participants in a field we were starting to see ourselves in.

We worked in places we might one day work in as professionals and began to imagine futures that hadn't seemed possible before. For me, CHOE connected the dots—it helped me realize that my place in healthcare wasn't just a dream. It was within reach.

Mrs. Meyer didn't stop there. She took us to the local community college, walked us through the halls, and introduced us to instructors. That college—where I first stepped foot as a high school student—would later become the place where I earned my associate degree in nursing science and teach as an adjunct professor of nursing years later.

I knew by then that I was on a path. And it all started because one teacher saw potential in me before I ever saw it in myself. Roberta Meyer taught me for three years. More than anyone else, she laid the foundation for everything that followed. She didn't just teach me how to prepare for a health career—she helped me believe that I belonged in one.

And through it all, my mother's voice stayed with me: *You can do what you want—as long as you earn that piece of paper*. That degree became more than a goal. It became a promise I made—to my family, to myself, and to every young person coming up behind me who might not yet see themselves in this profession.

Breaking Barriers

When I finally became a nurse, I quickly realized that being a Latino male in the profession came with challenges. Patients sometimes assumed I was a doctor instead of a nurse. Others questioned whether I had the knowledge or experience to provide their care. But I didn't let that stop me. Instead, I used those moments to educate, to break stereotypes, and to show that nurses come from all backgrounds.

I was born in Miami, Florida, and have lived in Washington, D.C., Tallahassee, New York City, and of course, D.C. again. Each place added another layer to my understanding of people and the role nursing could play in their lives. The diversity within the Latino community—from Caribbean to Central and South American roots—was reflected in every place I lived. That diversity has always been our strength.

As I gained experience, I felt a pull toward something bigger. I wanted to do more—not just for my patients, but for the next generation of nurses. That desire led me to further my education. After earning my Associate of Science in Nursing (ASN), I went on to complete my Bachelor of Science in Nursing (BSN), then a Master of Science (MS), and eventually a Doctor of Philosophy (PhD) in Nursing Research with a minor in Nursing Education.

The Power of Education and Mentorship

Furthering my education opened doors I never imagined. I taught at Miami-Dade Community College, New York University (NYU) Rory Meyers College of Nursing, and now at Georgetown University. I serve on boards of directors shaping nursing regulation and policy. I worked to make sure that more people—especially those from underrepresented communities—had access to quality education and real career opportunities in healthcare.

If there's one thing I've learned, it's that no one succeeds alone. I didn't get to where I am without mentors, and I've made it my mission to do the same for others. Whether through one-on-one mentorship, advocacy, or policy work, I've made it my goal to open doors for others.

Through my work with the American Association of Occupational Health Nurses and the Florida State Association of Occupational Health Nurses, I've had the privilege of helping to build pathways for aspiring nurses. I've also worked on initiatives to address nursing shortages in underserved communities, ensuring that future generations have the support and opportunities they deserve.

The Road Wasn't Always Smooth

One of the most significant challenges I faced during my career was navigating professional spaces where very few people looked like me or shared my background. There were moments of isolation, times when I felt I had to work twice as hard to be seen and heard. I've also experienced personal losses that shaped me—losses that reminded me of why this work matters and of the responsibility I carry for those who cannot speak for themselves.

What helped me through was community, culture, and that early grounding in family. Every time I faced doubt, I returned to my mother's voice, that mantra that became my compass. And I leaned into my purpose—not just to succeed, but to make space for others.

Looking Forward: A Legacy of Service

Today, I see Latinos reshaping the face of nursing. We bring our culture, our language, our families, our resilience. We understand our communities because we are our communities. Whether it's providing culturally responsive care, addressing health disparities and inequities, or leading the next generation of nurse educators and researchers—our impact is growing. And it's only the beginning.

My aspiration for the future? To continue reaching back. To serve as a bridge between where we are and where we're going. To create programs, policies, and pipelines that will elevate more Latinos into nursing and healthcare leadership. I want to continue mentoring, teaching, and shaping systems to be more inclusive and equitable.

Advice for Aspiring Latino Nurses

For those just starting their journey, here's what I want you to know:

Start where you are. Don't wait for the "perfect time." The first step matters most.

Find your community. Seek out mentors, organizations, and networks that will support and uplift you.

Own your story. Your culture, your background, your lived experience—they are assets. Bring them with you.

Get that piece of paper. Whether it's an associate degree, a bachelor's, or beyond—education opens doors.

Give back. As you rise, reach back. Always make space for others at the table.

A Lasting Legacy

Looking back, I see how far I've come—from the kid who never imagined himself in nursing to the mentor who now helps others find their way. But my story isn't just about me. It's about the people who guided me, the students I've mentored, and the future nurses who will continue to break barriers.

Success isn't about titles or awards—it's about making a difference. And if I've learned anything, it's that true success comes from reaching back and lifting others up.

That's the legacy I hope to leave behind.

Favorite Nursing Memory

One of my most defining nursing memories was caring for a patient living with HIV who used tincture of opium to manage severe diarrhea. He gently refused the dose I brought—it hadn't been prepared exactly the way he preferred. I wasted it, returned to the medication room, and remade it to his standard. It would've been easy to dismiss his request, but I realized this routine was the only part of his illness he could control. That moment shaped my practice and commitment to meeting patients where they are, honoring their autonomy, and delivering care that bears witness to their lived experience.

Biography

Rick García, PhD, RN, CCM, FAAOHN, FNYAM, FAADN (he/him/él), is the Chief Executive Officer of the Organization for Associate Degree Nursing (OADN) and the OADN Foundation. He continues to mentor aspiring Latino nurses across the country.

Rick is a dedicated nurse leader, educator, and advocate whose journey into nursing began in a high school health science classroom in Miami, Florida. The son of hardworking Cuban parents, Rick was the first in his family to earn a college degree—fulfilling his mother's mantra: *You can do whatever you want, as long as you earn a piece of paper that shows the world you went to college*. That piece of paper became four degrees, including a PhD in Nursing Research with a minor in Nursing Education.

Rick's dissertation examined the intersection of cultural competence among nursing faculty and the use of transcultural teaching behaviors in baccalaureate nursing programs in Florida. This work deepened his lifelong commitment to culturally congruent care through a lens of cultural humility—bearing witness to the lived human experiences of his patients, students, and colleagues.

Having lived in Miami, Tallahassee, New York City, and now Washington, D.C., Rick's career spans pointofcare nursing, academia, regulatory leadership, and national policy advocacy. As a proud Latino and openly gay man, he is committed to increasing representation and equity in nursing, especially for historically excluded communities.

In his free time, Rick enjoys traveling, taking daily long walks, spending time with his husband, family, and loved ones, and listening to live jazz at Mr. Henry's on Capitol Hill—where Roberta Flack was famously discovered.

You can connect with Rick at Rick_Garcia@mac.com.

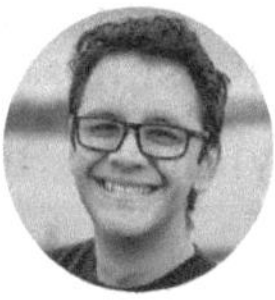

Pain Can Be Transformed Into Beauty; Share It With the World

DANIEL FELIPE MARTIN SUÁREZ-BAQUERO

"Take your broken heart, make it into art."
- Carrie Fisher to Meryl Streep

Current Position

I am an Assistant Professor at the School of Nursing at the University of Washington in Seattle.

What I Love About Nursing

What I love about nursing is its unique ability to turn pain—both our own and others'—into something meaningful. It blends knowledge, care, and artistry, allowing me to heal using my hands and my heart. In nursing, science, and humanity merge to create beauty even in the hardest moments.

Roots of Resilience

I was born during one of the most violent times my home country has faced: It was 1989 in Bogotá, Colombia, South America. 1989 was one of the most violent years in my country, marked by the crimes of drug cartels and criminal gangs. Fear was pervasive and permeated the lives of all Colombians. Car bombs, an airplane downed by a terrorist attack, the Medellín cartel — led by Pablo Escobar—controlling many aspects of national dynamics, and the assassination of Luis Carlos Galán, one of the most beloved candidates pursuing the Colombian presidency. These deep wounds, this violence, and this fear were going to shape my childhood.

Although this was the climate my country was embedded in, I grew up surrounded by women. There was my mother, the primary provider for a household of six; and my Abuela, who was always recognized as a healer.

My Abuela, Alicia, was an extraordinary woman. She taught me the power of plants, the love infused in cooking, the beauty of helping others, and the strength found in caring. My life was filled with dualities—the horror in the news contrasting with the warm protection of my Abuela's hands, the scent of her kitchen, and the kindness of her smile. I think she always saw me for who I truly was, without questioning why I preferred to be in the kitchen with her rather than playing with cars and fighting games with my brothers. She had the gift of reading souls, and she did read mine. My Abuela never finished elementary school, yet she was a quintessential nurse and midwife. She passed down to me the knowledge of healing, herbal remedies, caring for pregnancy, and catching and raising babies. I am sure her influence led me to become a nurse and a midwife.

Nursing, Academia, and the Fight for Recognition

I earned my undergraduate degree in Nursing from the Universidad Nacional de Colombia, and since these early stages, I have felt a deep passion for caring for childbearing women and pregnant-capable people. However, in a *machista* country like Colombia, this was troublesome. A male nurse specializing in maternity was scandalous. Maternity nursing was deemed a space exclusively for women. I heard comments like "How is a male nurse going to teach about breast-feeding, childcare, and newborn care? How can he catch babies at birth? Patients will feel uncomfortable." And yet, when it came to male obstetricians, their gender was never a problem. These obstacles led me to pursue a master's in nursing focused on Maternal and Perinatal Health. During my master's, I began to think more critically about our discipline.

Despite my deep connection to the core disciplinary nursing knowledge, I realized I couldn't see myself reflected in the faces of those White women who put themselves as dominating the field. I began to ask why my professors, and the great figures of Latin American nursing, were absent from these books. That's when I promised to bring our names, our voices, and our identities into the narrative, to reclaim our space in the history of nursing. I decided to become a nursing theorist, and to reveal the hidden dimensions of our profession, I had to go where those theorists were. That became my motivation to move to the United States to pursue a Doctor of Philosophy (PhD).

After more than ten years of clinical practice as a nurse and midwife, I arrived in the United States in 2018 to pursue my PhD studies at the University of Texas at Austin. When talking about Latin American nursing, the concept of *Cuidado* and the importance of traditional midwifery in my country as a means to reduce maternal mortality collided against the walls of academia like a speeding car crashing into a brick wall. I was told repeatedly that my research didn't matter, that Latin American nurses who focused on disciplinary nursing knowledge were irrelevant, and that traditional midwives should be integrated into Westernized healthcare systems.

These moments were all heartbreaking, and to be completely honest, I don't think my heart has ever been fully healed. It started getting sore when they bullied me when I was a child and a teenager for being gay, when my father and elder brother passed away, and when an older man raped me, made to feel guilty for who I was at the age of thirteen. He was just one of many men who have abused me throughout my life. My heart shattered when my grandmother left me. And now, it breaks again as I find myself feeling invisible, irrelevant, as an impostor.

It went far beyond impostor syndrome; my entire existence was being undermined by some of those reading my papers and hearing my voice as they said, again that my work and my thoughts were not important, academic enough, and a waste of time. I am deeply grateful for those few mentors who believed in me and supported my path, especially in the darkest moments when I thought of giving it all an end. Bullies have always been there. In the classroom as classmates, in the hospital as colleagues, and in academia as professors and mentors.

I took those pieces of my shattered heart and turned them into words. Art was my refuge when I was a child, I felt safe when singing, sewing, painting, and writing. As a nurse, I realized I could bring that into my science. I found a way to communicate my essence while contributing to reproductive justice and maternal health. That passion and determination led me to publish six papers from my dissertation and earn my Doctorate in Nursing Science—despite so many believing I wasn't enough.

That's how I secured a postdoctoral position at the University of California, San Francisco, and met one of the most incredible mentors and friends I could ever ask for. I don't even have the words to express my gratitude to the legendary Dr. Monica McLemore. She saw me, truly saw me, and believed in me. With her support, my career continued to grow, and now I am an Assistant Professor at the University of Washington School of Nursing in Seattle.

And yet, I still have to fight to prove that my work is important, that Latin American nursing is valuable, that traditional midwives must be protected, and that reproductive justice is a claim for human dignity and the most fundamental of human rights.

Reclaiming Space in Nursing

My work has inspired Latine nurses in the U.S., but more importantly, across Latin America. So many nurses feel seen through my words, and that is a true honor. My work has impacted Latin American nursing in ways I never imagined, it has made us question our identity in a field that was built and imposed upon us. There is something powerful in saying the names of so many invisibilized nurses in Spanish, standing before the American Academy of Nursing, and reclaiming our existence, our roots.

If there's one thing I've learned through my years in nursing, it's that there are many ways to make use of pain—of a broken heart, a shattered dream, a lost hope, the death of a loved one, or even the state of the world. Some create breathtaking paintings, some travel the world to find themselves, some dedicate their lives to helping others. But me? I have taken my broken heart and poured it into my words, my *Cuidado*, my pursuit of justice, and my fight to reclaim our identity as Latin American nurses. My articles are a crude reflection of my years in clinical practice, my search for knowledge in research, and my relentless pursuit of truth through the words and experiences of human beings. They have become, once again, a shout from the Global South, a shout for freedom.

We, Latines, are shaping the future of nursing by bringing our communities, our histories, and our lived experiences into the profession. We are challenging outdated structures, pushing for culturally responsive care, and advocating for policies that center our people, especially those who have been historically marginalized. Many of us come from families and communities where caregiving is second nature, where resilience is a survival skill, and where love is resistance. We take those lessons and turn them into action, whether by conducting research that centers the realities of Latine patients, fighting for reproductive justice, or mentoring the next generation of nurses who, like us, never saw themselves reflected in this profession. We are proving that science and care are not mutually exclusive, that knowledge comes in many forms, and that being a nurse is not just about what you know, but about how you show up for others.

Our success shows that you don't have to be born into privilege to make an impact. I never thought I would be where I am today—a professor at a prestigious university, a published researcher, a recognized voice in nursing. But I am here, not because the system made space for me, but because I carved it out. The next generation of Latines in nursing needs to see that there is no single path to success. Some of us come from working-class families, some of us speak with a "broken" English, some of us are first-generation college students who had to work multiple jobs just to get through school. Our presence in this field matters because it tells others: You belong here.

The most valuable lesson I have learned during my nursing path is that you don't need permission to take up space. For a long time, I felt like an imposter in academia, in nursing, in every room where people like me were not supposed to be. But the moment I stopped waiting for validation and started speaking my truth, everything changed. The greatest opportunity I've had is realizing that my perspective—my experiences as a third-world queer, working-class *sudaca*—brings something to nursing that no textbook ever could: My story, my art, my way of caring for others. That is my power.

I want to build spaces where nurses, especially those who have been excluded, can thrive. I want to decolonize nursing knowledge, challenge the hierarchies that define whose knowledge matters, and create pathways for others to step into this profession without having to erase themselves to fit in. I want to continue using art, storytelling, and qualitative research to disrupt the *status quo*. And above all, I want to ensure that nursing never forgets its Latin American roots—not just as a science, but as an act of love and resistance.

Critically, succeeding is not only a matter of perseverance, it is fundamental to find a mentor who understands your struggles and is committed to support your success. Also, we need to embrace our bilingualism and multicultural knowledge. When you start feeling like you don't belong, remind yourself: *El sistema no fue hecho para nosotres, pero igual aquí estamos*. You deserve to be in this field just as much as anyone else. Never forget to keep building community. Nursing can be isolating, especially when you don't see many people who look like you. Always remember why you started and where you are coming from, never forget your roots. There will be moments when you want to quit, when you doubt yourself, when the weight you are carrying is too much. Nursing is tough. But hold onto your purpose—either by fighting for health equity, representing your community, or simply by proving that you belong.

As I write this chapter, words move through me, waiting to take shape. To be true to oneself and to be valued for an authentic and meaningful life dedicated to making a difference is the greatest privilege of being a nurse. I am an artist, a nurse, and something beyond identity itself. My work, my art, and my nursing define my existence. My life is proof that pain can be transformed into care, into beauty, into something worth sharing with the world.

Nursing, art, love, and hope can bloom in the darkest moments. Many might say I am no artist, just a lucky *sudaca*. But who decides what it means to be an artist? Necessity forces creation. It pushes you to figure things out and to stop waiting for permission. That is exactly what I did with my life. Yes, I tried to end it. I have known sadness, the kind that lingers deep in the bones. But even in those moments, I sang, I painted, I wrote, and I dreamed. I imagined a different life. In the end, nursing and its relentless act of care saved me from everything I thought would consume me.

That world of elite nursing always felt distant, like a place I could never belong to. I have 19 published papers, a couple of book chapters, and I've lost count of the conferences I've spoken at; but even today, I still feel like an outsider in this world. I'm in a privileged position now. I became a professor at a renowned *gringo* university, but I know I don't belong, and I never will because I am a *sudaca* and a fagot from the lower social class. But now I am a *sudaca* they listen to.

I could never dream of having a spot in that imaginary line of nursing success, waiting for my turn. Ahead of me were nurses trained at prestigious universities in the North, fluent in English, who speak the language of science, use quantitative data, and run randomized control trials (RCTs), the ones who "really" know science. And you know what? I understand why they say what they say about me. Sometimes, I doubt myself too. I question everything I do. There are days when I think all my art and work are worthless—not just as an artist or a nurse, but as a person. I doubt everything because I was always told I wasn't good enough, and I believed it. But I keep moving forward.

The only thing I truly know is how to be an artist in nursing, to love this art of *Cuidado* that has saved my life, time and time again. Fear, that voice whispering that I am not enough, is nothing more than a wounded ego. But I have nothing to lose because everything has already been a gain; I have won against life itself. I share my nursing art with humility and with the deep respect that nursing deserves. Everything I create comes from the most primal part of my being. I am not here to take anyone's place, but I will never apologize for taking up my own.

Thank you to all the mentors who believed in me: *Mi Abuela* Alicia Vaca, *mi madre* Alcira Baquero, Martha Bejarano, Jane Champion, Loraine Walker, Lynn Rew, and Monica McLemore. I owe you everything I am.

Favorite Nursing Memory

I cannot choose just one favorite nursing memory—there are too many moments that have shaped me. I have helped bring hundreds of babies into the world, held hands of patients taking their last breath, offered hugs to comfort souls in pain, and witnessed tears of relief. I have also felt immense pride in uplifting my fellow Latin American nurses, reclaiming our space in the discipline. Every moment, from birth to death, from comfort to advocacy, reminds me why I chose this path. Nursing is not just a profession; it is a calling that transforms both lives and hearts.

Biography

Dr. Daniel Suárez-Baquero (he/él) is a Colombian nurse and Assistant Professor at the University of Washington School of Nursing. He earned his BSN and MSN from Universidad Nacional de Colombia and has over a decade of experience as a labor and birth nurse. He later obtained his PhD from the University of Texas at Austin.

Dr. Suárez-Baquero's work focuses on reproductive justice, qualitative research, and nursing theory. His research advances sexual and reproductive health care, particularly abortion access, through advanced qualitative methodologies. He is committed to decolonizing nursing knowledge and fostering equity in health care. He is actively involved in mentoring students, guiding research in nursing philosophy, and leading initiatives such as the UW ACTIONS program.

Beyond academia, Dr. Suárez-Baquero is an artist. He integrates painting, music, and sculpture into his perspective on nursing as both science and art.

He welcomes collaborations and connections via email at dmsuarez@uw.edu or on social media at @dmsuarezba.

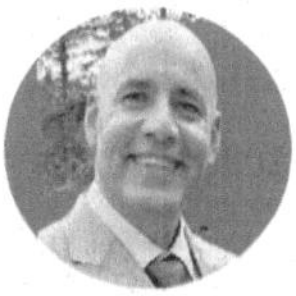

My Journey from Captain to Nurse

EDWIN DIAZ

"I think therefore I am."
– Rene Descartes
Father of Modern-Day Philosophy

Current Position

I am a Retired Fire Captain, Hartford Fire Department Engine 8, and a Registered Nurse in the Emergency Department, Vascular, and Endovascular Surgery.

What I Love About Nursing

Nursing is not simply a job; it's a calling. To embark on nursing, one begins a journey, learning skills, utilizing one's knowledge in order to benefit another. You are providing care to help one who is ill become healthy again. Nurses are impactful.

Intro to My Journey

One isn't raised to think they will leave behind a legacy or that they will be inspirational to others. I grew up in the Projects - Rice Heights (Hartford, CT). Typical kid, parents worked in factories for most of my youth. Father would become a CT Transit bus driver. I knew we didn't have money, but I didn't think of myself as lacking anything. I enjoyed my youth. The experiences I had early on gave me life lessons.

Let's divert to my earliest recollection of my interest in medicine. It comes from a tragic event. You see, I was hit by a car crossing the street when I was 5 yrs old (approx. 1975) which results in a Hip Spica cast during some of my kindergarten year. I had orthopedic visits with Dr. Elliot Sweet, a man I will always remember. He insistently encouraged me to learn, become educated, never work in a factory or with my body. "Become a lawyer, banker, doctor," he would say. These were his inspirational words to me each time I saw him in my follow up appointments. Early on those were frequent, then yearly, and well into my high school years. During those formative years, I would consider his words and those professions as my best options. I was truly enthralled with orthopedic surgery. So, if I were to pursue becoming a doctor, it would be nothing less than surgeon.

I recall constantly signing out a college anatomy textbook from the library at McDonough Elementary School. I would read it as best I could. I would intently study the pictures and diagrams of the body. This is probably the one and only book I enjoyed reading during my younger years. I was never a recreational reader. The Librarian would help me to understand what I read. Other students thought it was odd and gross, but I was intrigued with medicine and how one can heal from injury. Again, my event and Dr. Sweet bring this into focus for me.

I recall being given an aptitude test in the 5th grade. I'm not sure why, but I was scheduled to meet with the school counselor and the test administrator. She was the first person to ever tell me that I have a logical / scientific brain in the way I think, and problem solve; that I should aspire to become a scientist or doctor.

As a city kid with working class parents, how would I afford medical school? I did not know about scholarships, grants, and loans. Nonetheless, I was always drawn to the body, anatomy, science were strong subjects for me, especially things of medical nature. Dare I say, I was a closet nerd at a time when being a nerd was not a positive title to wear.

High school and definitely destined for college. Looking at a career path and landed on a goal: The Central Intelligence Agency (CIA), United Stated Drug Enforcement Agency (DEA), or The Federal Bureau of Investigation (FBI). I was also considering military service. However, military recruiters failed me. Each spoke of me enlisting and going into the Infantry. They would not speak to me about the Officer's track. I found their advice to be insincere. It seemed at odds to enroll into the infantry, serve several years and then pursue college and officer as a career if I could simply pursue the career upon enrolling. I would direct a recruiter to speak to me about careers such as Intelligence, Special Operations, or Pilot. As I aspired to join the CIA. I was firm to not become another statistic. One more Puerto Rican kid from the city becomes Infantry.

College Years

I was a strong B student, capable of doing more, but I did not do what was needed to get those As. The world I wanted was attainable with Bs and even in college, I did not embrace the nerdism.

Unbeknownst to me, life was leading me towards nursing. As an undergraduate, I was close to switching my major to nursing. Once I graduated, I worked for an insurance company. Like most companies at the time, they offered growth. I soon learned, in the corporate world, that growth is slow to come and was not my future path. I was actively pursuing law enforcement to get to CIA / DEA, was again considering the military. I remained motivated as I had flown down to CIA Headquarters for an interview. This was a great experience for me. It proved that my goal was attainable.

HFD—Hartford Fire Department

The Hartford Fire Department (HFD) was my landing spot. This was now my career and my path towards CIA - I would become a fireman and continue my quest. Then, the unexpected happened. I loved every part of being a Fireman. The life, the job, the brotherhood. After 2 years, I no longer looked towards the CIA. I focused on being a Fireman* and getting promoted to an Officer of some sort. * In 1994 this was the term, brotherhood as well. It slowly transitioned to Fire Fighter and Brotherhood / Sisterhood.

During my early years, we responded to medical emergencies despite little to no formal training for those types of calls. Yet, I always took to these calls as my youth and interest had prepared me for these incidents. Fast forward to today, there is formalized medical training at various levels. Emergency Medical Services (EMS) calls are now routine and an intrinsic part of every Fire Department.

Consciously, I was not thinking of nursing, but seems life was getting closer to it. Reality was promotions within HFD come slow. I evaluated my life and aspirations. Now with a family, I knew the CIA was ever so distant and unrealistic. I would never apply again. Retiring without a Plan B was also not my intent. Ergo, I was again bound for college. I self-reflected and landed on the "medical field." Slowly getting back to the interest I've always had since my youth. I eliminated becoming a Paramedic. I was already out in the field, once older I would not want to be outside in the snow, rain, or one more natural disaster. I knew whatever career I chose; it would be something within the hospital setting. If only I had become a Doctor, LOL.

Second Career Path, Now Closer to Nursing

My second career path would be Physician Assistant. I learned that Springfield College had a track. I applied and was given a list of 12 prerequisites courses I needed to complete before entering the program. I mapped this path out, attainable even while still being a firefighter. It would be years of school and hard work. Possibly even more than 10 years as I would do most parttime. Not once did I consider leaving HFD. No, I would pursue my Plan B, my second career, all the while being a Firefighter. I've got 10 years to get it done.

Serendipity

One Sunday, while my wife is reading the Sunday newspaper, serendipity steps in. I'm fully aware that this ages me in our modern-day world of tech. The University of Connecticut created an accelerated Bachelor of Arts to Bachelor of Science in Nursing (BA to BSN) program to help bridge the gap and have more nurses as the future predicts a shortage. An accelerated program is common today but not 20+ years ago. This was a novel program. I immediately applied, switching my mindset. Being a nurse was now my goal. I did not see it as sacrificing anything. It absolutely fits who I am, who I could become. Fortunately, I connected with a couple of administrators of the program and was given great encouragement and advice. I applied and was told of 6 prerequisite courses, and the program was 12 months. VERY DOABLE.

My realization at this point in my journey is that I always wanted and should have pursued a medical career. I would recall that anatomy textbook, Dr. Sweet's preachings, and now my life experiences as a firefighter. Nursing was absolutely a perfect fit for me.

1/9/09, Day 1 at the ER

January 9, 2009, I am a licensed Registered Nurse. I went to only one job interview with the Emergency Room at Hartford Hospital. I took the job that same day, at the very moment it was offered. Goal achieved and happiness attained. I was not daunted. I knew I would figure it out and learn nursing. Proudly, I can say, I'm also an excellent nurse. I possess talent, in some respects, and I possess skills. Fellow nurses can relate to these words and read within the line as this is not simply a job, but a calling. You cannot fake good nursing care. To anyone reading this, I hope you find it inspirational. Because any goal you set for yourself can be attained. Sometimes the path to that goal is straight forward, but other times, they are twist and turns. Life is not so easy, but it is absolutely worth living and making the sacrifices needed to achieve your dream.

Favorite Nursing Memory

Favorite Nursing memory will bring me right to my first clinical rotation within the hospital. My patient, Mary with her husband at her side. Initially ill but not considered critical. Mary was inquisitive and conversive. Soon after she shared her feelings and said that she would not be discharged. She was accepting that she would pass. Mary would always call me her angel and said that I brought her comfort. She felt God had sent me to her and it helped her accept and she transitioned and passed. I would also go on to be the nurse caring her Husband.

Biography

Edwin was born and raised in Hartford, CT. Early years lived in the Rice Heights section of the city. Then Frog Hollow neighborhood to the South End. He has a wife and three children.

Educationally always a good student, average or Bs but in high school several teachers encouraged him to do and try more. Honors classes were taken. Early on, he knew he would go onto college. Career aspirations towards something higher than himself. Top goal was the CIA (Central Intelligence Agency).

Life brought about opportunities and challenges. The first true career was HFD (Hartford Fire Department), and this is where Edwin developed his mindset and purpose in life. It was here within the culture of being a Firefighter in the city he grew up in and serving his people that Edwin blossomed. It was after a few years of serving that the thought of doing more sprouted. The next goal was set into place, and the journey began towards Nursing. It is the role Edwin currently enjoys as he has retired from HFD (June 1994 to June 2016) but remains an active nurse. He welcomes collaboration and connections via email at ltedrn@yahoo.com.

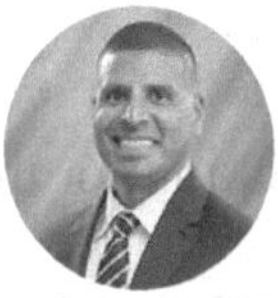

From Lima to Leadership: A Nurse's Journey of Resilience, Advocacy, and Impact

JIMMY A. REYES

"Be the change you wish to see in the world."
– Gandhi

Current Position

I am an Assistant Professor of Practice at the University of Northern Iowa and Proteus Interim Clinical Director.

What I love About Nursing

I love nursing for its profound impact on lives, the privilege of caring for others, and the ability to advocate for underserved communities. It blends compassion, science, and leadership, fostering lifelong learning and resilience. Nursing allows me to empower patients, mentor future professionals, and create meaningful change in healthcare.

My Personal Journey

I was born in the vibrant city of Lima, Peru, and spent my formative years surrounded by the warmth of family and the rich cultural heritage of my homeland. My roots also extend to Chile, where my parents' stories of resilience and determination shaped my early worldview. Growing up in a bicultural household meant that celebrations were a blend of Peruvian and Chilean traditions, with food, music, and community playing central roles. This early exposure to diversity instilled in me a deep respect for different perspectives and an appreciation for the strength found in unity.

Some of my earliest memories as a child growing up in Chile are of my grandmother, Violeta, who was a home health nurse. She would often take me to work with her and the interactions she had with her patients will forever be etched in my mind. She cared for each of her patients as if they were family, and it is because of her that I wanted to become a nurse. My grandmother's selfless dedication left an indelible mark on my heart, guiding me toward a path of compassion and service.

My journey to the United States began at the age of 16 when my parents emigrated in search of better opportunities. We settled in Saint Cloud, Florida, where the contrast between our vibrant Latin American culture and the new, unfamiliar environment was stark. Adapting to a new language and culture was challenging, but it also fueled my determination to succeed. I quickly realized the importance of education and community in creating a sense of belonging and purpose.

The Motivation to Become a Nurse

My decision to become a nurse was deeply influenced by my grandmother's example and my early experiences of caregiving within my family. I vividly remember accompanying my grandmother to medical appointments and attending community events. These moments ignited a passion in me to bridge the gap between healthcare providers and patients from diverse backgrounds. I wanted to ensure that others, like my grandmother, could receive compassionate and culturally competent care.

Determined to pursue a nursing career, I moved to Iowa in 1999 to attend the University of Iowa College of Nursing. I was drawn to its outstanding nursing program in gerontology- a passion I developed after observing my grandmother care for the elders in her community. While pursuing my education, I worked at a local hospital, gaining valuable clinical experience and reinforcing my commitment to the nursing profession.

Now, 25 years later, I am still in Iowa, dedicated to advancing healthcare, supporting underserved communities, and mentoring the next generation of healthcare professionals.

Success in Nursing

One pivotal moment in my career came during a particularly busy shift at the hospital. A nurse practitioner encouraged me to apply for the John A. Hartford Predoctoral fellowship. This program designed to address the shortage of nurse educators and promote diversity, provided financial and professional support to full-time minority students enrolled in graduate nursing programs. The opportunity was like a springboard for my career. Thanks to the scholarship, I completed my graduate education at the University of Iowa College of Nursing and embarked on a path that combined clinical practice, education, service, and research.

Today, I am a nurse educator, practitioner, and advocate for underserved and underprivileged communities and populations. I have also developed my own program of research related to the management and prevention of Diabetes Mellitus Type 2 among older Latinos in rural areas. These roles have allowed me to contribute to the profession in meaningful ways, shaping the next generation of nurses and addressing critical health disparities.

Biggest Challenges and Losses

One of the most significant challenges I faced was navigating the healthcare system as an immigrant and a first-generation college student. There were moments of self-doubt and feelings of being an outsider in a field that lacks representation from individuals like me. Also, the loss of a close family member during my early career tested my resilience and reminded me of the fragility of life. This personal loss deepened my empathy for patients and their families, reinforcing my commitment to providing holistic care.

Overcoming Obstacles

The obstacles I encountered—both personal and professional—were daunting, but they became stepping stones toward growth. During my graduate studies, I collaborated with other nursing, pharmacy, and social work students to open a migrant health clinic. We balanced class in the mornings, clinic work during the day, and evening visits to care for agricultural workers in rural areas, often staying until midnight. These experiences were challenging, but they solidified my passion for serving underserved populations.

I relied on the support of mentors, family, and community to navigate challenges. Connecting with other Latino/a nurses provided a sense of camaraderie and shared purpose. Professionally, I sought opportunities to develop my skills and advance my education, earning advanced degrees that opened doors to leadership roles. These experiences taught me the importance of resilience, adaptability, and the power of a strong support network.

Diversity Within the Latino/a Community

The Latino/a community is incredibly diverse, encompassing a wide range of cultures, languages, and experiences. This diversity is both a strength and an opportunity to create meaningful change in nursing and healthcare. As a Latino nurse, I am proud to represent this vibrant community and to advocate for equitable healthcare access. My work with underserved populations has shown me the profound impact of culturally competent care and the importance of amplifying voices that are often unheard.

Shaping the Future of Nursing

Latinos/as are playing a pivotal role in shaping the future of nursing by bringing unique perspectives and a deep understanding of cultural nuances to the field. Our presence in leadership positions and our commitment to addressing health disparities are inspiring the next generation of nurses. I believe that by sharing our stories and creating pathways for others, we can continue to break down barriers and build a more inclusive healthcare system.

Inspiring the Next Generation

To aspiring Latinos/as in nursing and healthcare, my message is simple: Believe in your potential and seek out opportunities for growth. Surround yourself with mentors and advocates who will champion your success. Remember that your unique background and experiences are assets that enrich the profession. Together, we can create a more equitable and compassionate healthcare system.

Valuable Lessons and Opportunities

One of the most valuable lessons I have learned is the importance of embracing change and viewing challenges as opportunities for growth. Each step of my journey has been marked by moments of uncertainty, but these moments have also been the most transformative. The opportunity to mentor and inspire others has been a profound privilege, and I am grateful for the chance to contribute to the advancement of nursing.

Future Aspirations

Looking ahead, my aspirations are to continue advocating for health equity and to expand access to education and resources for underserved communities. I envision a future where every aspiring nurse has the opportunity to thrive, regardless of their background. By fostering collaboration and innovation, I hope to leave a lasting impact on the profession and the communities we serve.

In conclusion, my journey from Peru and Chile to a fulfilling career in nursing has been marked by resilience, determination, and a deep commitment to making a difference. I am proud to be part of a profession that values compassion, diversity, and lifelong learning. Together, we can continue to shape the future of healthcare and inspire the next generation of Latinos/as in nursing.

Favorite Nursing Memory

One of my favorite nursing memories was during a migrant health clinic visit in rural Iowa. An elderly farmworker, hesitant at first, shared his struggles managing diabetes due to language barriers and lack of access to care. After patiently explaining his condition in Spanish and providing culturally relevant education, his eyes lit up with relief. Months later, he returned, proudly showing improved blood sugar levels and expressing deep gratitude. That moment reinforced my passion for serving underserved communities, reminding me that nursing is not just about treating illness, it is about building trust, empowering patients, and making a lasting difference.

Biography

Jimmy A. Reyes serves as the Interim Clinical Director at Proteus and a faculty researcher at the University of Northern Iowa. He brings extensive expertise in nursing education, regulation, health policy, and research focused on underserved and low-resource communities.

He holds advanced degrees in nursing and gerontology, including a PhD from Concordia University Chicago and a Doctor of Nursing Practice from the University of Iowa. His research focuses on culturally anchored, family-centered programs aimed at improving diabetes self-management among Latinos, particularly in Federally Qualified Health Centers. Additionally, he facilitates diabetes self-management research in Yola, Nigeria.

Jimmy has held diverse leadership positions including Project Director at the University of Iowa, Associate Director of Practice and Education at the Iowa Board of Nursing, and Dean of Nursing at Kirkwood Community College. He remains actively engaged in advancing public health initiatives.

He welcomes collaborations and connections via email at Jimmy.reyes@myhealthiowa.org or on social media at linkedin.com/in/jimmyareyesphddnpagnprnfreaa051224.

[illegible]

[illegible] serves as [illegible] Internal Clinical [illegible] Director [illegible] reaches the [illegible] Ministry of [illegible] education [illegible] [illegible] language [illegible]

He holds a [illegible] degrees in nursing and [illegible] including a PhD [illegible] concentration [illegible] and a Doctor of Nursing Practice from the University of Iowa. His research focuses on culturally anchored, family-centered programs aimed at improving diabetes self-management among Latinos, particularly in Federally Qualified Health Centers. Additionally, he [illegible] diabetes self-management research in Yuma, [illegible]

He has held [illegible] leadership positions including [illegible] Director at the University of Iowa, Associate Director of Practice and [illegible] at the Iowa Board of Nursing and Dean of Nursing at Kirkwood Community College. He remains actively engaged in advocating public health [illegible]

He [illegible] social [illegible] family [illegible] health [illegible] [illegible]

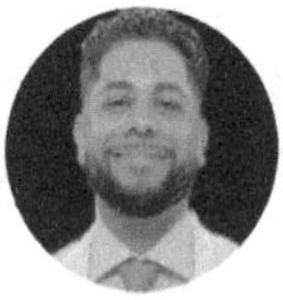

Nursing Wasn't Always For Me, or I Didn't Think It Was

OSCAR DANIEL BAHENA

"Develop success from failures. Discouragement and failure are two of the surest stepping stones to success."
– Dale Carnegie

Current Position

I am a New Graduate Nurse in the Neurosciences Intensive Care Unit at the flagship hospital for one of the major health systems in Chicago.

What I Love About Nursing

Nursing is versatile. There is so much more to nursing than working in a hospital or clinic. We can go into the community to vaccinate to prevent the spread of diseases, we influence policy to improve healthcare and even address global health challenges and health disparities. The options are limitless.

Mi Historia

Nursing wasn't always for me, or I didn't think it was. Since eighth grade, I knew I wanted to be a veterinarian –I LOVE animals, so that was the goal to achieve. However, life has taken me through a journey in both my personal and professional life that led me to where I am today (and it is definitely *not* what I had planned), but I've made it work, and I truly feel this is where I am supposed to be.

Mi Trayecto

I was born in Chicago to a Puerto Rican mom and Mexican father. After I finished kindergarten, my family moved to Puerto Rico where we lived until I completed seventh grade. In Puerto Rico, we lived *en un monte* on the east side of the island *en el pueblo* known as Naguabo. We were surrounded by so many trees and cool animals like snakes, lizards, and birds. I would catch the snakes and lizards to keep as pets and sometimes brought home stray dogs. This is where my love of animals began. Moving back to Chicago was a shock–there was no more greenery and no more nature. In eighth grade we were asked to write a paper about what we wanted to be when we grew up. To be honest, I hadn't thought about it because things didn't move that quickly in Puerto Rico. This assignment took some time, but that's when I decided to be a veterinarian.

Throughout my high school career, I was laser focused on achieving that goal. I got into the University of Wisconsin-Madison (UW) where I would major in animal science. Unfortunately, I dropped out after completing sophomore year because my family could no longer afford to send me to an out-of-state school. I foolishly declined admission to local schools that offered scholarships when UW did not, all because I wanted to major in animal science—I had a plan, but I did not have a backup.

¿Enfermería? ¡¿Por Qué?!

After dropping out of school, I had to work and that's when I eventually found a job as a filing clerk at a small law firm that focused on medical malpractice. This jump-started my career in law where I worked my way up to paralegal. During my 12 years in this role, I served clients from diverse backgrounds, particularly those from underrepresented communities, providing them with competent and compassionate support during their most difficult times.

My decision to go to nursing school was initially to supplement my paralegal career as I wanted to start my own business and break away from law firms. I continued to work for my employer a year into nursing school until it became apparent that I could no longer balance the two while doing good work in both. After quitting, I took advantage of as many opportunities in school as I could get my hands on. It was this semester where nursing school made a huge impact on my life. Unsurprisingly, this was also when I was taking my community course and started working as a graduate assistant in community-based research.

During March 2024, the new arrival migrant community in Chicago residing in shelters throughout the city experienced a measles outbreak (CDPH, 2024). As part of the UIC Outbreak Response Team (ORT), in partnership with the Chicago Department of Public Health (CDPH) and other healthcare providers, we went into the shelters to offer, administer, and educate about vaccinations and illness. After nearly three months, the measles outbreak in Chicago was officially over (CDPH, 2024)!

From my time in this setting, I recall one gentleman on a day that I was working an 8-hour shift. It was mid-day, and he refused to be vaccinated;his wife and children received the Measles, Mumps, and Rubella (MMR) vaccine earlier. I spoke with him and asked what prevented him from getting the vaccine. He told me they had been poked way too many times since first arriving in the

U.S. Of course, who wants to get a needle stuck in them that many times?? While I understood, I explained that the shelter where they were staying was for families and there were pregnant moms and babies that could not get the vaccine. This meant it was up to everyone else that could get vaccinated to get it for the protection of the vulnerable. I saw in his eyes he was thinking about it but hadn't yet made up his mind. Several times he walked into the room we were in, then walked back out. No kidding, we had about 20 minutes left in our shift, and he came in again. I asked what he decided. He said he wanted the vaccine. This was a huge win, and I felt so proud of myself. Maybe I could do this nursing thing.

In addition to the previous experience, my community-based clinical rotation required us to enter the Cook County Department of Corrections (CCDOC), where we engaged in health promotion efforts addressing subjects that the detained individuals expressed a desire to learn more about, such as stroke, prostate cancer, attention-deficit/hyperactivity disorder (ADHD), depression, etc. To that end, we developed educational handouts, oral presentations, and interactive activities to create positive spaces for the learners.

Seeing that the majority of the incarcerated people looked like me was eye opening, to say the least. As of this writing, roughly 70% of detainees in the CCDOC identify as Black while about 20% are Latino (CCSO, 2025). In comparison, the Black and Latino residents in Cook County were estimated to account for 23.6% and 26.3% of the population, respectively (U.S. Census Bureau, 2023). Meanwhile, White individuals accounted for a substantial 65.1%. When comparing the Cook County figures to those of the CCDOC, the total percentage of Black and Latino residents reaches almost 50%, significantly lower than the White demographic in Cook County (U.S. Census Bureau, 2023). During this experience I kept thinking: "I could have easily been one of them and they could have been my shoes. What was the difference and where was the bifurcation in the road that led us to be where we were?" This got me to deeply consider the intersection between the criminal justice system and social determinants of health, and the potential for incorporating restorative justice to improve the lives of detainees before, during, and after incarceration.

Mi Motivación

When we returned to Chicago from Puerto Rico, I was in eighth grade and what a blow that was. My brother and I were frequently taken out of class to be tested on our English competency, despite not showing any deficiencies in our ability to read, write, or speak English. We were performing well in school overall. The challenging part was math. I remember in seventh grade we were studying fractions;adding, subtracting, etc. Somehow, I got an A in the class. Coming to Chicago, I was severely behind in math. I think they said I was like at a fourth or fifth grade level; so much so that I did not remember how to do anything with fractions even though I did it the year prior. I thought I was going to fail and be held back. I remember one of my cousins telling me I "better not fail because no one in our family has been held back." I felt that burden to do well.

Luckily, my math teacher had a passion for teaching and was great at it, albeit, strict. He used a math program that was adaptive to our learning. If we got concepts right, it would give us more challenging problems and/or moved us up to a harder level–if you took the National Council Licensure Examination (NCLEX), you know what that's like. I can't tell you how helpful this program was. I advanced 4 to 5 grade levels in a matter of one year!

School here was completely different from what I was used to in Puerto Rico. In Chicago, we apply to high schools in eighth grade, but since recently moving from PR, I didn't know anything about them. In Puerto Rico we just went to our pueblo's escuela superior in tenth grade, unless we went to a private school. I went to open houses and the high schools are enormous here! I had only seen these types of schools in movies. There was one high school I wanted to attend because I was told it was good for math and science. Unfortunately, I missed the deadline to apply and was required to enroll in my neighborhood school, which had initially rejected my application. Fortunately, I was somehow accepted into the International Baccalaureate (IB) program and was allowed to take Advanced Placement (AP) classes all throughout high school. To be completely honest, I don't think I belonged there. Everyone was so smart, and they knew stuff. I was just learning and trying to keep up.

For as long as I can remember, I was expected to go to college; there was no question about it. I was supposed to behave and get good grades. The tradeoff, I didn't have to work, so that's what I did–I got the good grades, had the high GPA, was at the top of my class. I was the model student…or, so I thought. Come senior year, I had come to terms with something about myself that I had been confused about for years–I was gay. I came out to my family, and I did not get the "warm welcome" I thought I would receive. All my efforts and hard work in school did not matter now and the main focus was my sexuality. I was kicked out of home, and various times left to fend for myself. My grades suffered and my class ranking dropped from #4 to #9. While I was still in the top 10, I knew I wasn't at the top of my game, even with everything going on. I would stay late in school to apply to colleges, writing my application essays and personal statements. I still had to meet expectations.

Going to UW was challenging. I was away from home surrounded by people that did not look like me. I was not used to this. I recall receiving an email from a student organization for "students of color." What the heck was that? Was *I* a student of color? I had never in my life until that point been referred to a "something" of color. It made me feel different. Was I meant to be there? The pressure of being on my own, struggling with my sexuality and my experience the previous year caused me to go into a depression to the point of having suicidal ideations and planning. I went to counseling to figure out how to properly deal with my emotions.

Obviously, I didn't follow through with my plans. In the face of all these challenges, I had a feeling I was meant for something. Life didn't take me where I wanted, but I ended in fields where I focused on helping people experiencing one of the most difficult moments in their lives. Whether I am a paralegal or nurse, I am making a difference and I know this is what I am supposed to be doing.

Favorite Nursing Memory

During my community clinical, I shadowed a home hospice nurse to visit her patients. Our first patient legit lived across the street from the barbershop where I got (and still get) my haircut. We weren't in this house for more than a few minutes when the patient passed away while doing our assessment. The family was Spanish-speaking, and the nurse wasn't, so it fell on me to talk to them and provide comfort. I had never seen someone die before and it took everything in me not to cry. I will forever carry that experience and its emotions with me.

References

- Chicago Department of Public Health (CDPH). (2024, May 30). Health Alert. Measles update: *End of Out-break declaration*. https://www.chicagohan.org/alertde-tail?p_p_id=hanalertdetailsweb&p_p_lifecycle=2&p_p_state=normal&p_p_mode=view&p_p_resource_id=download&p_p_cacheability=cacheLevelPage&_hanalertdetailsweb_attachmentId=45704759&_hanalertdetailsweb_priv_r_p_alertId=46684778
- Cook County Sheriff's Office (CCSO). (2025, February 28). *Sheriff's Daily Report*. https://cookcountysheriffil.gov/wpcontent/uploads/2025/02/CCSO_BIU_CommunicationsCCDOC_v1_2025_02_28.pdf
- U.S. Census Bureau. (2023, July 1). Quick Facts: Cook County, Illinois. https://www.census.gov/quickfacts/fact/ta-ble/cookcountyi llinois/PST045223

Biography

Oscar Daniel Bahena, MSN, RN, is a Registered Nurse in Chicago. He earned his Master of Science in Nursing from the University of Illinois-Chicago in 2024. Prior to pursuing a career in nursing, Oscar dedicated over a decade to the legal field as a paralegal, focusing on various matters, including personal injury, medical malpractice, and civil rights. Oscar's previous experience informs his nursing practice by providing him with a uniquely holistic perspective when interacting with his patients.

Oscar was born in Chicago and is of Mexican and Puerto Rican heritage and descent. At a young age, his family moved to Puerto Rico where he spent his elementary school years. This exposure helped him cultivate a strong bond with his Puerto Rican culture and community. Returning to Chicago for high school, Oscar resettled in his old neighborhood on the city's Northwest Side.

His combined experiences give him a passion for working with underrepresented populations. He plans to attain higher education to positively impact underserved communities, locally and globally.

He welcomes collaborations and connections via email at odbahena4@gmail.com or on social media at IG: oscarit0_o [zero underscore littleO].

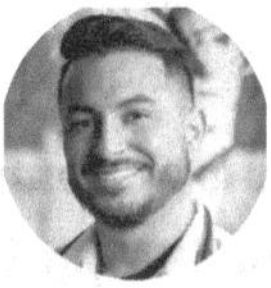

Sigue Adelante:
A Neurodivergent Latino Nurse's Journey of Breaking Barriers

LUIS ALEJANDRO ROLDÁN CUBIDES

"We do not wait for change; we create it. We break barriers, build bridges, and open doors for those who come after us."

Current Position

I am a Nurse Practitioner and an Adjunct Nursing Faculty.

What I Love About Nursing

Nursing is more than a profession; it is a commitment to healing, advocacy, and empowerment. It means standing beside patients in their most vulnerable moments and ensuring they feel seen and heard. As a Latino neurodivergent provider, I use my unique perspective to challenge systems, advocate for equity, and transform healthcare for all.

A Journey of Resilience: From Colombia to the United States

I was born in Colombia, a country known for its spectacular landscapes, rich traditions, and a strong sense of community rooted in family values. In our culture, family is at the heart of everything. No matter the challenges, we lean on each other to move forward. However, the 1990s brought great uncertainty. At the peak of the cartel war, many communities faced violence and instability. My mother wanted to provide me with a better future, so she moved us to the United States.

Securing a visa was no easy task. The process was filled with obstacles, uncertainty, and no guarantees. But when our approval came, we knew this was our chance. I arrived in the United States at eight years old on Halloween night, October 31, 1997. I completely forgot it was Halloween night, and I recall seeing people in costumes at the airport and thinking, "So this is how things are in America." Amid my excitement and anxiety, I had no idea how much my life would change.

I did not speak English and knew no one in this country. Due to the language barrier, I had to repeat the third grade. School became overwhelming and intimidating, but I reminded myself that my mother sacrificed everything for me to have this opportunity. However, being the only person of color in a predominantly Caucasian school made me feel isolated and different. I was often treated differently, and for the first time, I experienced shame, guilt, and not belonging. As I moved through middle and high school, challenges continued to mount. Each time I encountered difficulties, I was often told to "try harder," “focus more,” or “pay attention." I tended to rush through assignments, completing them quickly but making mistakes due to not thoroughly reading the instructions. I always felt several steps behind, yet I was determined to hide my struggles from others. At home, failure was not an option; my mother had made too many sacrifices, and I could not disappoint her. There was no room for poor grades.

I often felt like I was never enough. No matter how difficult it was, I learned to mask my struggles and pretend I belonged because I could not risk letting anyone see how hard I was fighting to keep up. Despite these challenges, I recognized that education was the key to a brighter future. I did not just want to succeed for myself; I wanted to help my family and honor my mother's sacrifices.

Overcoming Barriers: My Path into Nursing

I always knew I wanted to help others, but I was uncertain of the path. During college, I became a certified nursing assistant (CNA) and discovered my passion for patient care. Being at the bedside, aiding patients, and witnessing the dedication and expertise of nurses reassured me that this was my destiny. Nurses were caregivers, advocates, educators, and the essence of healthcare. Navigating college as an immigrant student was daunting. I struggled with the Free Application for Federal Student Aid (FAFSA) without the proper support while managing academic expectations. When I applied to my first nursing program, the director suggested I explore other career options. I vividly recall sitting in her office as she told me that nursing was not the right field for me. That moment could have destroyed my confidence, but instead, it ignited my resolve. Having already overcome numerous challenges, I was determined not to let one person's viewpoint dictate my future.

At home, I faced another challenge. When I told my mother I wanted to become a nurse, she questioned why I was not becoming a doctor. In Latino culture, nursing is often seen as a female-only profession, and in some countries, it does not carry the same prestige. But I knew that nursing was my purpose. The more I learned about nurses' impact, the more I understood that this was where I could make the greatest difference.

That part of my life marked a low point. I felt overwhelmed, exhausted, and uncertain about why I could not keep up despite my efforts. I sought counseling, and through that process, I was diagnosed with attention deficit hyperactivity disorder (ADHD). For the first time in my life, things began to make sense. Suddenly, all the years of being told to "try harder," the constant forgetfulness, the inability to regulate emotions, the racing thoughts, and the frustration with traditional study methods—it all finally had a name. Accepting my diagnosis was not just a relief; it was transformative. It allowed me to stop blaming myself, start learning more about my brain, and try the right medication to help me be the best version of myself. Understanding my ADHD helped me rewrite my narrative. I stopped seeing my mind as something to fix and started honoring it as a source of creativity, resilience, and insight.

Despite my passion, my journey to nursing was not straight-forward. When I recognized that nursing was my calling, I had already accumulated too many credits to change majors, so I completed my bachelor's degree in biology. However, I refused to let that deter me. I applied to a different nursing program at another university. This proved to be the best decision I could have made. The program was accelerated, running year-round with only one week off in the summer and one in the winter. The intensity challenged me academically and personally, reinforcing my passion for nursing. Within 18 months, I earned my Bachelor of Science in Nursing (BSN) - Registered Nurse (RN), a milestone that felt both hard-earned and immensely fulfilling. This experience shaped me into a more resilient, adaptable, and dedicated healthcare professional, readying me for the next phase of my journey. After a few years of working as a nurse, I was inspired by other nurses and nurse practitioners, so I applied for a master's program to become a family nurse practitioner. While working full-time as a nurse, teaching clinical part-time, attending school part-time, getting married, buying a house, and having a baby, I graduated successfully in three years with my master's and became a family nurse practitioner. I have loved doing it and continue striving to improve patient care daily.

A Nurse's Impact: Representation, Neurodiversity, and Advocacy

Becoming a Latino nurse, a neurodivergent provider, and a parent to neurodivergent children has given me a unique perspective on healthcare, education, and advocacy. As a nurse practitioner, I do more than treat illnesses; I educate, advocate, and ensure every patient feels heard and valued. Many of my Latino patients tell me they have never had a provider who looks like them, speaks their language, or truly understands their struggles. As a neurodivergent provider, I know what it is like to navigate a system that was not built for my brain. I ensure that neurodivergent individuals receive compassionate, personalized, and effective care. I also reflect on my struggles as a child, how I masked my difficulties and felt like I had to fight to keep up. As a parent of neurodivergent children, I now advocate to ensure they do not have to struggle as I did. My spouse and my kids, who are also neurodivergent, inspire everything I do. They remind me why inclusivity in healthcare and education is so important.

In addition to my work as a provider and parent, I have found community through the Greater Milwaukee Chapter of the National Association of Hispanic Nurses (GMNAHN). I have been a member since its founding in 2018 and had the privilege of serving as a board director. Being part of GMNAHN has been empowering; it is a space where I feel supported, uplifted, and understood by colleagues with similar experiences and backgrounds. I am forever grateful for their presence in my in my life and their role in helping me get to where I am today. Seeing more nurses who look like me and actively lead change in our community is powerful and inspiring.

Final Thoughts: Creating *Nuestra Mesa*

For too long, Latinos have been excluded from leadership in healthcare. But when no one offers us a seat at the table, we build our own. We create nuestra mesa—a space where we uplift, mentor, and support each other, ensuring that future generations face fewer struggles than we did.

To my Latino and Latina colleagues in nursing: *Sigue adelante*. We need you, we see you, and we are here for you.

And remember, we belong here.

Favorite Nursing Memory

One of my most unforgettable nursing memories was caring for a patient with advanced heart failure who eventually received a left ventricular assist device (LVAD). I first took care of him as a CNA and later as a nurse, witnessing his long battle while waiting for a heart transplant. Over time, we developed a deep friendship. The day after Valentine's Day, he received the call for his new heart and personally called me to share the news. Although I was not working, I visited him on the unit and brought heart-shaped treats to celebrate this life-changing moment. The following day, he was in the ICU, and the nurse who was caring for him called my unit to let me know that he asked for me. He had a special request. I went to see him and congratulated him on his new chance at life. I wondered if he had listened to his heart yet, and when he shook his head to say no, I handed him my stethoscope. When he heard the beat of his new heart for the first time, he started crying, and so did I. It was a moment of hope, resilience, and second chances I will cherish forever.

Biography

Luis Alejandro Roldán Cubides, MSN, APNP, FNPC, (he/him/él), known as Alejandro, is a Latino nurse practitioner, educator, and advocate for neurodiversity and health equity. Born in Colombia, he immigrated to the United States at the age of eight, overcoming language barriers and systemic challenges that ignited his passion for advocacy and patient-centered care. Despite facing discouragement in pursuing nursing, Alejandro remained determined, demonstrating that obstacles are meant to be surpassed. As a neurodivergent provider, he leverages his lived experiences to promote inclusive healthcare, empower underserved communities, and confront inequities within the system. His dedication extends beyond patient care; he is also an adjunct nursing professor, inspiring the next generation of nurses to lead with compassion, cultural humility, and purpose.

As a parent to neurodivergent children, Alejandro is deeply committed to promoting mental health awareness and improving access to neurodiversity in healthcare and education. His work is grounded in the belief that representation is important and that every patient, regardless of background, language, or neurodivergence, deserves to be seen, heard, and valued. Through his career and advocacy, Alejandro is dedicated to paving the way for future generations, ensuring that Latinos in healthcare have a seat at the table and the opportunity to create their paths.

He welcomes collaborations and connections via email at npalejandroo@gmail.com or on social media @Npalejandroo on TikTok & Instagram and YouTube: Nurses Unidos.

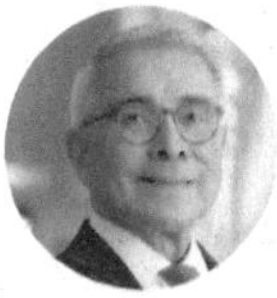

Breaking Barriers and Inspiring The Next Generation of Nurses

ELIAS PROVENCIO-VASQUEZ

"To succeed you need to embody the true spirit of perseverance and passion."

Current Position

I am a Dean and Professor for the College of Nursing at the University of Colorado Anschutz Medical Campus.

What I Love About Nursing

It is a chance to make a difference in people's lives.

Introduction

Over the past 40 years I have been a practitioner, educator, administrator, and researcher. As a clinician I practiced as a neonatal/pediatric nurse practitioner. I entered academia full-time after many years as a neonatal nurse practitioner (NNP) and was appointed director of the NNP program at University of Texas (UT)-Houston Health Science Center, School of Nursing. I maintained an active role in teaching in undergraduate and graduate nursing programs until I was appointed Dean in 2010.

Since 2010, my primary teaching activities have been at the doctoral level. The varied administrative experiences throughout my professional career have helped me bridge practice, education, and research efforts with real world needs. These efforts are supported by meaningful collaboration, innovation, data-informed decision making, reasoned risk-taking and the astute alignment of resources and objectives. As a researcher, I am well known nationally and internationally for my work with "at risk women and men." The overarching focus of my program of research is to reduce health disparities, in Hispanic/Latino women and men, related to substance abuse/use, intimate partner violence and high-risk sexual behavior.

Since 2010, I have served as Dean of University of Texas at El Paso School of Nursing (UTEP SON). Our vision for UTEP SON was to become a leader in nursing practice, education, and research in the global healthcare environment. Our commitment to diversity is interwoven into the academic, research, and service mission of our SON. With a minority student population of 80%, UTEP is designated as a Hispanic-Serving Institution. During my tenure, the school doubled enrollment, which stood at 1300 students, the highest in program history. New academic degree programs implemented during my deanship include a Doctorate of Nursing Practice (DNP) and a Psychiatric-Mental Health Nurse Practitioner Program (first cohort, spring 2018).

Other leadership experiences I have had include being former President for the American Academy of Nurse Practitioners; Director of the Neonatal Nurse Practitioner program at the University of Texas-Houston and University of Maryland Baltimore; Associate Dean for Academic Affairs, Associate Dean for Undergraduate Programs and Associate Dean for Community Affairs at the University of Miami School of Nursing and Health Studies. In addition, I have also served on national panels such as the Task Force on Education and Regulation of Professional Nursing Practice for the American Association of Colleges of Nursing; the National Advisory Council on Nurse Education and Practice, Health Resources and Services Administration; and on the Finance Committee for the American Association of Colleges of Nursing. I am a fellow in several prestigious national organizations: United States Public Health Service Primary Care Policy Program; Robert Wood Johnson Developing Leadership and Reducing Substance Abuse; American Association of Colleges of Nursing Leadership for Academic Nursing Programs; Robert Wood Johnson Nurse Executive; American Academy of Nurse Practitioners; and American Academy of Nursing.

Teaching

Drawing from my experiences as a prior student, teacher and now mentor, my teaching philosophy is grounded in two central themes: the value of education and power of grit. Based on personal and academic perspectives, I have experienced the power of education on social mobility, health, and wellbeing. As stated by Horace Mann, "education is the great equalizer." Through the life experiences of students, I have witnessed that grit (passion and perseverance) is crucial to achieving the highest levels of academic and personal goals. For these reasons, when I interact with students, I help them envision the end goal that education, plus hard work, will help them achieve. I am convinced that student success is strongly influenced by a clear appreciation of the value of education and the power of grit.

To inspire students, I approach every teaching opportunity with the intention of engaging, challenging, and developing student knowledge. I am also convinced that students become enthusiastic learners of health, the impact on healthcare outcomes, or any other subject, when actively engaged in vivid exploration of relevant theoretical, experimental, or practical frameworks. For the past twenty-five years, I have had extensive teaching experiences and responsibilities across undergraduate and graduate nursing curriculum in didactic, online, and clinical settings. These teaching experiences have been cultivated in different settings in academia (University of Texas-Houston, Rutgers The State University of New Jersey, University of Maryland-Baltimore, University of Miami, and University of Texas at El Paso). My personal commitment, driven as a first-generation college graduate, is to enhance access and excellence in public higher education for all has never been stronger.

Mentoring

Despite my administrative responsibilities as Dean, I help educate and mentor the next generation of health disparities researchers and practitioners, through Doctor of Philosophy (PhD) and DNP courses. I am committed to mentoring under-represented minority students. Since my appointment as Dean in 2010, I have mentored doctoral students from various disciplines. For example, I have chaired or served on the dissertation committee of 12 PhD students (4 in nursing and 8 in interdisciplinary). Eleven of the 12 were under-represented minority PhD students. I have also served as chair or committee member for 5 DNP capstone projects, including one from Duke University.

Scholarship

My goal as a nurse scholar is to reduce health disparities through excellence in research. I have made significant contributions to health disparities science focusing on underserved populations, specifically "at risk" women and men of Hispanic/Latino descent. My program of research focuses on the intersection between substance use/abuse, intimate partner violence and high-risk sexual behavior. I continue to collaborate with a research team from the University of Miami, School of Nursing and Health Studies (UM SONHS). As a team, we have published and presented in nursing, community, and interdisciplinary forums, nationally and internationally. We have published in a breadth of journals to include nursing, sexuality research and social policy, men's health, social service, cultural diversity and ethnic minority psychology, gay and lesbian social services, men and masculinity, sexuality and culture, and Hispanic Health Care International.

Clinical Practice

Throughout the mid-90s, I practiced as a neonatal/pediatric nurse practitioner at the K.I.N.D.E.R. Clinic (Kids in Need of Drug Evaluation and Rehabilitation). I provided primary care to infants exposed prenatally to drugs, alcohol, and HIV. During this time, the nation was facing a growing number of mother-to-child transmission of HIV and the so-call "crack babies." My practice identified that not only were these exposed infants at risk, but so were their mothers. In response to this concern, I developed a model program for neonatal nurse practitioners to provide home visits to these high-risk infants and their mothers. The intent of these home visits was to support and empower mothers to parent their high-risk infants/children. I led a team of 5 neonatal nurse practitioner students to deliver 500 home visits to mothers with a substance use disorder, over a 4-year period. This work resulted in the development of red flags during home visitation for at risk infants and children. 26 Red flags are any physical, developmental, or psychosocial findings identified during a home visit that require further evaluation or referral. I also authored a chapter, in a maternal child nursing textbook, related to community and home care nursing for the high-risk infant.

Scholar

I learned from my clinical practice that mothers were the gate keepers for their children's health and well-being, therefore my research focus shifted to women at risk. Women at risk for substance use/abuse, intimate partner violence and high-risk sexual behavior. I was Co-Primary Investigator (PI) on Project D.Y.V.A. (Drugs and Violence in the Americas) funded by the Inter-American Drug Abuse Control Commission. Subsequently, I received funding, and was PI, for several funded research projects; Packaging Project SEPA: A Proven HIV Behavioral Inter-vention for Use with Latinas at Highest Risk of Acquiring HIV (CDC); Project VIDA (Miami): Violence, Intimate Relationships, and Drugs among Latinos (NIH) and Project VIDA II (El Paso): Violence, Intimate Relationships, and Drugs among Latinas/os (NIH). As I continued to develop my program of research, in collaboration with a research team at UM SONHS, our work expanded to address and reduce health disparities among women and men of Hispanic/Latino descent.

Academic Leadership

My academic leadership career began in 1993, when I was appointed director of the NNP program at UT-Houston School of Nursing. I then moved on to lead the NNP program at the University of Maryland School of Nursing. As the result of my leadership abilities, I was recruited to the University of Miami School of Nursing and Health Studies and was appointed Associate Dean for Academia. As enrollment increased, I transitioned into the role of Associate Dean for Undergraduate Programs. The experience gained from these appointments positioned me to be a successful transformational leader at UTEP SON. As Dean, I led and have final responsibility for the SON's curriculum and degree/certificate programs, faculty appointments, research and scholarship and community engagement. I continuously examine healthcare trends and workforce projections to modify programs or develop new programs to meet the needs of the changing healthcare landscape- I frequently ask myself, what will healthcare look like in five years. I provided visionary leadership to promote and foster research and scholarship in a SON committed to teaching and practice.

As the result of my academic leadership, I have served on the Task Force on Education and Regulation of Professional Nursing Practice for the American Association of Colleges of Nursing; the National Advisory Council on Nurse Education and Practice, Health Resources and Services Administration; and the Finance Committee for the American Association of Colleges of Nursing. I am a fellow in several prestigious national organizations: United States Public Health Service Primary Care Policy Program; Robert Wood Johnson Foundation in Developing Leadership and Reducing Substance Abuse; American Association of Colleges of Nursing Leadership for Academic Nursing Programs; Robert Wood Johnson Nurse Executive; American Academy of Nurse Practitioners and American Academy of Nursing.

I was involved in national healthcare reform initiatives; I served on three Robert Wood Johnson Foundation advisory committees - all supporting the implementation of the Institute of Medicine recommendations for the *Future of Nursing*. As Chair of the Doctorate Advancement Nursing Committee, I led a group of academicians developing an action plan to promote doctoral education in nursing. The other two committees included the Tri-Council for Nursing, advancing state and regional strategies to create a more highly educated nursing workforce and New Careers in Nursing, expanding nursing student capacity in accelerated baccalaureate programs. I served on two national organization committees: Governance Committee, American Association of Colleges of Nursing and Minority Fellowship Program National Advisory Committee, American Nurses Association.

I have worked with national organizations throughout my academic career that include: member of the research committee for American Academy of Nurse Practitioners and Association of Women's Health, Obstetric and Neonatal Nurses; grant reviewer for Substance Abuse and Mental Health Services Administration and Health Resources and Service Administration; American Academy of Nursing (AAN) Expert Panels on Violence, Health Disparities and Substance Abuse/Mental Health; committee member for AAN fellow Selection Committee; Mentor for the Ethnic Minority Fellowship Program for the American Nurses Association; and Ad Hoc panel reviewer for the National Institute of Child Health and Human Development, National Institute of Nursing Research-Special Emphasis and Nursing Science for Children and Families, Risk Prevention and Health Behavior-Special Emphasis Challenge Grants (2002-2009). I am currently a member the Minority Fellowship Program National Advisory Committee, American Nurses Association, and the National Governance Committee for the American Association of College of Nursing.

Summary

In summary, I have made significant contributions to practice, education, academic leadership, and scholarship. I have been very fortunate to have had opportunities to mentor and teach many students and faculty colleagues, to explore innovative ways to deliver care and to increase their understanding of health disparities and atrisk communities. One of my greatest strengths, as an academic leader, is that I relate extremely well with people from many different backgrounds and know that it takes a lot of people to make a winning team. My record of scholarship contributes to decreasing health disparities and improving health among women and men of Hispanic/Latino descent.

Favorite Nursing Memory

Throughout the mid-90s, I practiced as a neonatal/pediatric nurse practitioner at the K.I.N.D.E.R. Clinic (Kids in Need of Drug Evaluation and Rehabilitation). I provided primary care to infants exposed prenatally to drugs, alcohol, and HIV. During this time, the nation was facing a growing number of mother-to-infant transmission of HIV and the so-call "crack babies." I developed a program for neonatal nurse practitioners to provide home visits to these high-risk infants and their mothers. I led a team of 5 neonatal nurse practitioner students to deliver 500 home visits to mothers with a substance use disorder, over a 4-year period.

Biography

Over the past 40 years, Dr. Provencio-Vasquez has been a clinician, educator, administrator, and researcher. He is well known nationally and internationally for his work with "at risk women" and their families. He is an experienced neonatal and pediatric nurse practitioner. His background and expertise are in primary care and developmental assessments of HIV and drug exposed infants, children, and adolescents. Dr. Provencio-Vasquez is a pioneer in creating innovative nursing approaches (home intervention) for mothers with substance use disorders and their children.

His leadership experience includes being former President for the American Academy of Nurse Practitioners; Associate Dean for Academic Affairs at the University of Miami; Director of the Neonatal Nurse Practitioner program at the University of Texas-Houston; and University of Maryland-Baltimore. Dr. Provencio-Vasquez is a former Fellow with the Robert Wood Johnson Nurse Executive Program. He holds fellowship status in several prestigious national organizations: United States Public Health Service Primary Care Policy Program; Robert Wood Johnson Foundation in Developing Leadership and Reducing Substance Abuse; American Association of Colleges of Nursing Leadership for Academic Nursing Programs; Robert Wood Johnson Nurse Executive; American Academy of Nurse Practitioners and American Academy of Nursing. He welcomes collaborations and connections via email at eli.provencio-vasquez@cuanschutz.edu.

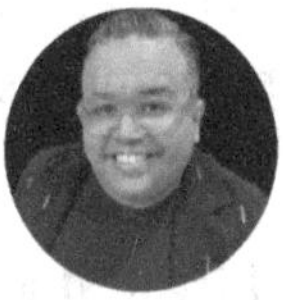

A Chicano's Nontraditional Journey into Nursing

ADRIAN ESPINOSA

"Un Dia A La Vez"

(Unknown)

Current Position

I am a Family Nurse Practitioner working at a Federally Qualified Health Center.

What I Love About Nursing

There is a unique and distinct connection that comes with the responsibility of being a nurse. Providing care and sharing space for diverse walks of life, while being able to make a special connection with patients who identify with me, is a privilege that I do not take for granted.

Building Community & Identity

In late spring of 2012, as I was completing an intense, accelerated year of nursing school, I found myself sitting next to my Tia Modesta in the emergency room. Little did I know that it was just a few weeks shy of her leaving us physically during a valiant battle with metastatic cancer. As we shared these sacred moments, it led us to an important promise. I promised my Tia that I would always treat my patients as I would want my family treated in the hands of a healthcare provider. This was important to both of us, after witnessing both the compassionate and callous sides of healthcare.

I grew up in the heart of East Side San Jose (ESSJ), raised by two hard working Mexican parents that migrated to the United States (U.S.) as young adolescents. They raised my sister and I with a strong sense of community and respect for a strong work ethic. Growing up, I loved visiting my Abuelita Paulita "Mama," who sparked an innate curiosity within me, as I tried to understand why she was injected with a liquid substance, drawn up from a glass vial, multiple times throughout the day. To this day, the smell of insulin reminds me of her and this life saving medication. Growing up in ESSJ during the 90s, I had my first introduction to chronic conditions resulting in amputations, domestic violence, teenage pregnancy, and a heavy gang presence. As I began to gain perspective on how social determinants of health affected my neighbors, I also felt a strong sense of resiliency throughout my neighborhood and the communities I began to identify as home. This is where I learned that I identified as not only Latino, but a Chicano; a first-generation Mexican American.

My parents enrolled me into a medical magnet high school to help nurture my aspirations of entering the medical field. When it came time to apply to college, I was fortunate enough to be accepted into multiple universities in other cities that had strong premed programs, but financially my family and I were not prepared for the steep cost of relocating plus tuition. From the age of 15, I had worked at our local Tropicana shopping center to help save for college and this afforded me the opportunity, along with my parents' support, to attend our local San Jose State University (SJSU). This is where the true complexities of academia and identifying my journey came into fruition. I found myself unprepared for challenging courses in the premed sciences, intimidated by the mere thought of approaching a professor for support. Even scarier for me during the late 90s, was sitting in a large classroom with very few folks that looked like me, wondering if they could tell that I had been born "different" as I found out early in puberty that I was attracted to the same sex.

My Nontraditional Road into Nursing

The journey of self-discovery throughout my undergraduate years at SJSU involved being proactive in finding a support system that I could relate to as an ethnic minority, majoring in the sciences and being the first in my immediate family to attend college. No one introduced me to other disciplines in healthcare other than medicine. Nursing was not a field that many males in a Latino household were being encouraged to pursue. During my time at SJSU, I came across a Chicano professor with his PhD in Chemistry, named Dr. George Castro. His mentorship ended up changing my life and helped serve as a catalyst that motivated me to continue my journey. Dr. Castro introduced me to Chicanos/Latinos in Health Education (CHE) and encouraged me to take on leadership positions while offering employment at his science workshops with youth looking for afterschool activities in some of the toughest neighborhoods. This era also blessed me with opportunities to meet lifelong friends and colleagues of Latino backgrounds, who were sprinkled throughout the colleges of science, nursing, and health science.

As I worked hard to build a career and foundation based on advocacy, service, healing and community building, there were moments that became challenging while living "closeted" in a career path that often entails sharing our own vulnerabilities. I recall taking a health education course, in the midst of a heavy load of science courses, with Dr. Kathleen Roe, a professor with a thirst for community health and a passion for teaching. What made her even more impressionable was that she was a white woman, well versed in culturally proficient practices, and had a genuine desire to uplift the next generation of diverse (in every essence of the word) public health leaders. This interaction and experience via the health sciences culminated into a perfect storm, as I solidified my goal to complete a Bachelor of Arts in Biology with a double minor in chemistry and the health sciences. After completing my undergrad, I later applied to the highly respected Master of Public Health (MPH) Program, with an emphasis in community health education in 2005, also at SJSU.

Acceptance of My Two Spirited Identity

For the first time in a while, I had direction. I knew that I wanted to create a fusion between public health and clinical practice and began to learn about various disciplines that afforded this opportunity, including nursing. Just as my professional and academic journey began to make sense, our family experienced the devastating loss of our matriarch - my Abuelita! Recognizing how short and precious our time on Mother Earth is, I decided it was time to embrace my identity and shared with my parents and select loved ones that I no longer saw myself as "different" but born the way that I was created through love and a higher power. This was pivotal in my late 20s, as I was blessed to receive the validation that I had yearned for, when I began to identify as a member of the LGBTQ community.

My personal development flourished as my professional development led me to work for schoolbased health centers, as a health educator and later a health education manager. These roles involved collaboration with multidisciplinary teams and included primary health care providers (PCPs), including nurse practitioners (NPs). Witnessing the autonomy and opportunity to provide care for patients while incorporating the spirit of nursing resonated and seemed to fill in a missing puzzle piece. Yet, the nursing world was still new to me, and I had to explore this exciting profession, heavily dominated by women with very few Latinos that I could look up to.

Evolving as a Latinx Nurse Leader

It was important for me to apply to nursing schools in California, as I knew I wanted to invest my training towards the communities of the Bay Area. I was fortunate enough to be accepted into the University of California, San Francisco (UCSF) School of Nursing, which had a Master's Entry Level Program for applicants who had a previous bachelor's degree. Stepping foot into class on the first day of nursing school at a top-rated program brought me great pride, with a touch of disbelief. I made sure I obtained the appropriate academic resources I needed to succeed, based on my learning needs, and moved to the city of San Francisco so I could focus and commit the next four years of my life training as a nursing professional.

Being one of the few males and Latinos in my program, I became involved with a newly formed campus organization named "*Voces Latinas*," where I shared space with a small but strong network of peers who made me feel at home away from home. I was also introduced to the National Association of Hispanic Nurses (NAHN) where I began to get involved with my nursing community at a larger scale and eventually grew the Greater San Jose Chapter's membership and later served on the national board of directors.

The training and clinical experiences I completed during my years at UCSF allowed me to value the time commitment needed to care for others, while learning the delicate balancing act of quality time with loved ones. My faith reminded me that I had to remain resilient if I wanted to contribute to the less than 7% of Latinos who made up the nursing workforce. To this day, I am confident that my familia's love, the support of my village, and my Tia Modesta's spirit, all walked me across the stage at graduation when I finally completed my nursing training.

From my first job as a Registered Nurse (RN) and subsequently as a Family Nurse Practitioner (FNP), my heart and commitment remained unwavering, as I sought employment at county and federally qualified health centers (FQHCs). Navigating the complex healthcare systems where multigenerational families continuously face countless barriers to healthcare, was a challenge that I wanted to contribute solutions towards. For approximately five years, I worked both as an RN and FNP, which provided variety in my routine and the income to begin putting a dent in my student loans. This overlap was becoming a heavier workload and then the Covid-19 pandemic hit. This was a daunting era that challenged me physically and emotionally. It was exceptionally painful losing colleagues and loved ones, while also witnessing and experiencing the harsh reality of bullying and racism within the nursing profession.

Becoming My Biggest Advocate in The Nursing Profession

Through the toughest of times, we find our greatest allies and strength. I began to observe the high demand at community clinics, as society began to return to some normalcy, post Covid, therefore I decided to focus on working at one FQHC as an FNP. During this time, I also renewed my faith in the supportive outlet that my diverse, Latino nursing familia could provide. The pandemic and combined experiences of other inspiring nursing professionals brought insight that identified a need to create additional safe spaces for the nursing community where we could address topics of incivility within the profession, while empowering our next generation and current nursing workforce. The universe aligned and I embarked on a lifelong mission, as one of the co-founders and current president of the Society of Latinx Nurses (SOLN). SOLN was born in 2022, from the vision of five inspiring nurse leaders and countless stories among our extensive nursing community.

Your Voice

Finding your voice will come at different times throughout your professional and personal journey. I have dedicated my life towards mentoring and increasing visibility for the nursing workforce while highlighting the needs of nurses of color. As a community, we still face cultural, financial, and institutional barriers that are challenging to navigate, especially when one may feel alone in a sea of faces that do not look like our own. During this journey, it is important to document your story. What may feel as the road less traveled, is actually the path that more peers need to hear about and identify with. In addition, remember to surround yourself with individuals who uplift, celebrate, encourage, and cheer YOU on. This circle becomes smaller over time, but it is a space that will keep you grounded while inspired to continue on your journey of service. I have learned that at the end of the day, I will not remember someone based on their extensive credentials at the end of their name, but by how they treated others.

I do not take for granted the privilege of providing care and bringing communities together. My padres Francisco y Guadalupe sacrificed so much so that my sister, Erica, and I could dream and succeed. As a proud son of immigrants, I honor the roots that have cultivated and flourished the Mother Earth that I walk on today. As my story only continues to be written, I take moments to remind myself of my Abuelita's (Mama's) philosophy to live life, "*Un Dia A La Vez*" (One day at a time).

Favorite Nursing Memory

My favorite nursing memories continue to transpire when I most need to hear them. Seeing the glow on a patient's face as they proudly share their accomplishments when reaching their A1c (three-month blood sugar average) goal, lowering their blood pressure, or reaching a specific health goal. Reminding patients that they did the work, while providing me with the privilege to walk alongside them for support is priceless!

Biography

Adrian is the proud son of Mexican immigrants. His parents began working in the agricultural workforce of the Salinas Valley in the late 70s, with the hope of providing both he and his sister an opportunity to excel in life and academia. After graduating from the public school system, Adrian attended San Jose State University (SJSU), where he completed a Bachelor of Arts in Biology (2004) and subsequently a Master of Public Health (2007). He later returned to nursing school and trained as an advanced practice nurse at the University of California, San Francisco (UCSF) (2011-2015). While at UCSF, he was selected as one of the Madison Clinic Peggy Huang Diabetes Nurse Fellows in the School of Nursing. In 2019, he received the *Signature Award for Service* from Northern California's Kaiser Permanente Latinx Association (KPLA). In 2020, Adrian was recognized as a *2020 UCSF campaign Alumni Awardee* in "The Pathfinders" category, as well as a "40 Under 40: Rising Nurse Leader" and completed a two-year term (2021-2023) as the UCSF

Nursing Alumni Association President. Most recently, he cofounded the Society of Latinx Nurses (SOLN) in 2022 and is the inaugural president.

He welcomes collaboration and connections via email at adrianmph@gmail.com and solnursesofficial@gmail.com and on social media @adrianelenfermero and @solnurses.

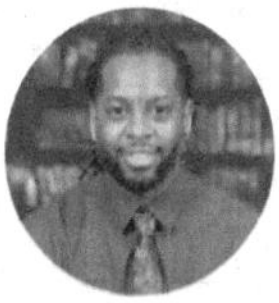

Quizas Algun Dia o Un Espacio para Ti

MICHAEL WILLIAMS

"In this profession, you can be jaded, but you should never be bored. There is always somewhere new to explore."

Current Position

I am a Nurse Practitioner providing at-home wellness exams, Visiting Clinical Assistant Professor at a University, and board member of a men's health clinic and of a national nursing organization, DNPs of Color.

What I love About Nursing

Nursing has allowed me to explore areas of humanity that are often overlooked and develop my sense of creativity through the art of caring for others.

"Quizas Algun Dia" is a motto and guiding principle I developed as an undergraduate student. It is a way for me to speak to my inner child—the first-generation American Afro-Latino Brooklyn boy who watched the world in amazement and wondered what the future held.

It is a reminder of my Panamanian mother, who would wake me up on Saturday mornings to the smell of *Hojaldres*, bacon, eggs, and *crema de maiz*, the sound of salsa, the warmth of love, and reserved pleasures of house cleaning duties. To understand my nursing journey, you should understand one thing about my mother: she never allowed me to stray away from the path that was mine. Before I left home for college, I had many lessons on accountability, peer pressure, and the consequences of allowing others to dictate your journey. Once I left the comfort of home, I realized English was different from the one I learned in my community, and standardized testing did not care about the cultural nuances of my upbringing. The nursing profession talks about culturally competent care but often forgets to include these considerations in their academic programs for students.

While my nursing career has been met with many challenges, the most pivotal moment occurred in my first year of nursing school. I struggled academically and internalized it as a lack of ability to learn, but my nursing faculty advisor changed that perception with her insight into my academic struggles. She told me my poor performance on exams and quizzes had nothing to do with my intelligence, and it was heavily due to cultural reading comprehension. She recommended I learn standardized English and how to take exams, removing my sense of imposter syndrome and validating my cultural uniqueness. My mind reframed the perceived shortcomings as an external task and not an inherent deficiency in my humanity. I still failed my initial pathophysiology course and spent the rest of my undergraduate life walking on a tightrope. Despite the immense distress of the "two failures and out" policy, I found time to engage in my community through service and social gatherings. Something I was told would hinder my success as a nurse because it took away time from nursing, but in my heart, being an active part of the community was a key element of nursing. To effectively navigate the program's pitfalls, I had to seek shelter and support from those outside the profession. This constant reminder helped develop my approach to care, which has carried over into my practice as a doctoral-prepared nurse practitioner. Aspects of who I was as a person – long locs, sneakerhead, regular use of slang, first-gen American, and college student were things that others viewed as barriers to my professional success. But those perceived barriers were precisely the things that allowed me to excel in nursing.

Leverage Your Uniqueness

At all levels of the profession, the patients we serve value trust, meaningful care, authenticity, and respect. Being a bilingual nurse and showing up authentically proved extremely useful as an inpatient medical-surgical and Trauma ICU RN. My walking into a room surprised many, but once we engaged in storytelling and allowed patients to see the person caring for them, I received the unspoken nod of approval and trust. My realization of the importance of who I was and represented to the community became more apparent as a Nurse Practitioner working in Internal Medicine at a Federally Qualified Health Center in Connecticut.

Speaking Spanish, understanding the nuances of various Latin cultures, and tapping into my lived experiences from growing up in a dynamic space like New York City positioned me to connect efficiently with those I care for. To be a Nurse Practitioner is to have regular access to some of the most vulnerable, raw, and unique aspects of the human experience. I'm not defined by the degrees I possess but by my life's journey, so my approach to care is ensuring my patients understand that I'm part of the community and not above it. Promoting conversations from favorite sneakers and anime to health and social inequities facing our Black and brown communities enhances the importance of another key principle of mine. Improving the health of our community is wealth-generating, a potent form of advocacy, and an essential bridge to reducing health inequities.

Disruption is Part of Your Existence

The Latino Nursing voice is powerful, and our presence is essential to the profession's advancement. Knowing when to utilize your voice and presence together or separately is crucial. The work required to transform nursing and healthcare into a more equitable space for the Latino community must be multilayered with explicit and passive resistance.

I learned very quickly that some of my white colleagues had a difficult time accepting me outside of the nursing framework. I passively challenged preconceived notions of professionalism through my hairstyles (inspired by Busta Rhymes), pairs of kicks like Jordan 1s or Asics GEL-Lyte III, and my Panamanian pendant - Ojo de Venado. Questions such as "Why are you speaking like that?" (referring to my use of slang) or "How can someone be here all these years and not know English?" were uttered by white individuals I had great relationships with who did not see me for who I indeed was and held a projected version of Mike. To those questions, I would reply with something like, "You don't need to speak perfect English to thrive if you have community," " You know Jesus spoke in parables, right?" or "Many of the people I view as great human minds spoke in rhymes." Slang, for me, is not a fad or part of some outfit I wear to authenticate my Blackness with patients - it is my language, along with Spanish and English.

Bring All

As a first-generation American college graduate, the road to becoming who I am was uncertain. Despite strong family and social support, the journey felt like I was a foreigner in a new land with many moments of loneliness and isolation. Those moments live vividly in my mind and motivate my academic engagement as a clinical professor. My goal is not to produce better nurses but to create an environment that fosters better humans who are more cognizant and appreciative of their influence as nurses. To show an example of blending professionalism and being true to oneself. Creating a space where accents and other cultural nuances can thrive because the clinical environment allows students to take their knowledge from lectures and apply it to human experiences.

Our Collective Duty

I'm Black. I'm Latino. I'm beautifully Panamanian-made and Brooklyn-raised. My parents always forced me to explore the meaning of my true self and instilled a great appreciation for the small, often overlooked steps in life that define our legacy. It is within these small steps that Latino nurses are and will continue to transform the profession. I'm here today because of the many people who invested parts of their lives into mine, and with that comes a cost. The cost is my duty to the collective: to share knowledge, invest in others, and make way for the future until I no longer exist. We are not asking others to share our stories and spaces. We are not asking for permission to enter spaces that we are more than qualified for. We are taking them, adding flavor, and bringing others with us. In the words of Christopher "Notorious B.I.G." Wallace, "Spread love that's the Brooklyn way." Words I live and practice as a nurse practitioner.

Favorite Nursing Memory

As an inpatient medical-surgical RN, I was approached by a patient who planned to get married in the hospital, and the couple requested that I walk her down the aisle. She was a patient that I had cared for frequently over the years, and on this admission, lasting several months, her prognosis was unfavorable. Our unit and the chaplain service assisted in successfully executing the wedding. To be considered and to play such a role in a special occasion was humbling. Despite the patient eventually passing away, her memory lives on with me.

Biography

Dr. Michael Williams (He/Him) is a board-certified Advanced Practice Registered Nurse (APRN). As a bilingual (English, Spanish) APRN who specializes in Internal Medicine and HIV-PrEP, he has provided care to a culturally and socioeconomic diverse patient population for over seven years. Along with clinical practice, Michael has been a clinical instructor at several institutions.

Michael believes community care is essential to the advancement of society. The philosophy guiding his practice is to provide the highest level of care through meaningful and collaborative relationships with all community members. As a first-generation college graduate, he and four friends initiated an endowment scholarship for first-generation college students at their alma mater.

Along with philanthropic efforts, he engages in various speaking and volunteer events in his community. He has been featured on Telemundo Austin for World AIDS Day, highlighting the importance of STI/HIV testing and prevention in the Latino population. He has also been featured in the Wall

Street Journal to discuss the increase in males pursuing nursing careers. Michael firmly believes that improving healthcare outcomes begins with educating and empowering the community he serves. He welcomes collaborations and connections via email at mwill0614@gmail.com and via social media at @soleofaNP and https://www.linkedin.com/in/michaelwilliamsdnpaprnfnpbc85a870123/.

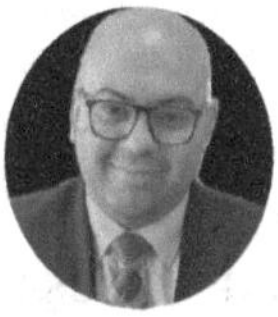

Unmoored, Yet Homeward Bound

ZAFAR ANWAR

"Pies, ¿para qué los quiero si tengo alas para volar?"
– Frida Kahlo

Current Position

I am an Assistant Professor at Columbia University's Doctor of Nursing Practice in Nurse Anesthesia Program and Certified Registered Nurse Anesthesiologist for an anesthesia service in a quaternary medical center.

What I love About Nursing

What I love about nursing is the quiet privilege of being there—when a person is most vulnerable, when their world has unraveled. To serve in those moments, to offer care, steadiness, even the smallest comfort—it is an honor. Sometimes, all we can do is witness. Sometimes, that is enough.

Chapter 1: Humble Beginnings

When I cast my mind backward through the fog of memory, I do not see a straight path but a crooked lane paved with the coarse cobblestones of hardship, love, and longing—a path shrouded in the mist of time and illuminated only by the occasional lantern of joy. The first flicker of light: my father's silhouette at JFK Airport, his presence breaking the spell of years spent apart. He had arrived in America in the early 90s—a time when the word "immigrant" carried both aspiration and accusation—working three jobs, sleeping on borrowed couches, sending home money with more care than he gave himself, all so we could one day follow.

And we did. The day we boarded the plane remains half-shrouded in nausea—my airsickness was legendary—but clearer is the memory of anticipation, an ache in my chest shaped like a continent. Excitement and dread danced together in uneasy truce. We landed, the pressure in my ears giving way to the relief of arrival, and there he stood, waiting. Years vanished in a single embrace.

Our first American meal was a kind of sacrament: McDonald's, Filet-O-Fish, fries pooling in one shared heap on a paper plate. We sat cross-legged on the cold floor of a bare Brooklyn apartment, the walls still smelling faintly of someone else's life. Yet even there, among boxes and echoes, it felt like home.

Brooklyn in 2004 was a city of collisions: of cultures, dreams, subway delays, and the incessant hum of becoming. At nineteen, I walked its cracked sidewalks with the brittle confidence of the newly arrived. I claimed my piece of it in the classrooms of college and through my activism with New York Public Interest Research Group NYPIRG,that odd little acronym that stood for something much larger—service, equity, voice. I was learning to speak, not just in English, but in purpose. I also learned to speak through a stutter I had carried for much of my life. With NYPIRG, I learned how to stand in front of rooms and advocate, even when my voice shook. That shaped me.

But then October came, and everything unraveled like a poorly tied shoelace. My father—my anchor, my compass—was gone. It was not cinematic, just a quiet absence that stretched into forever. That night, I sat beside my mother as her silence gave way to sobs, her body trembling like a tree refusing to fall. Time blurred. Mornings and evenings lost distinction. In the dark, I whispered promises I didn't yet know how to keep.

In that shadow, I found my first thread of resolve: I would be the man of the family now. It was a role I didn't know how to play, but grief is a stern teacher.

Nursing found me not like a revelation but like an echo—an echo that only made sense after it passed through me. When my mother was diagnosed with stage IV lung cancer, I saw—truly saw—what nurses could do: not just tasks, not just charts, but dignity amid despair. They carried stories, not just syringes. They translated chaos into comfort.

I transferred to Hunter College, grasping at the edges of certainty. My first clinical experience was humbling. A fellow student and I stumbled through the choreography of a bed bath, awkward and apologetic. Our elderly patient chuckled at our ineptitude, then guided us with the kindness of someone who had made peace with their own frailty. When we finished, his gratitude was incandescent.

That evening, the sun dipped low and generously, gilding the city in amber. Standing there, scrub top damp and heart full, I knew. This was it.

And then—again—the ground shifted.

Undocumented." "Illegal." Words that always seemed to hover around someone else's story now branded mine. With my father gone, my visa was void. I was placed in removal proceedings. My future—the white uniform, the stethoscope, and the humble pride of care—became a mirage.

Two years in bureaucratic purgatory followed. I was depressed and afraid. Each sunrise arrived with dread; each trip to the mailbox felt like a blade. I wasn't sure what my future would hold. I just hoped—sometimes blindly, often desperately—that something would work out. If it didn't, I would've had to pivot. I didn't know how. But thankfully, I never had to.

Then came court: a narrow room that smelled of mildew and resignation. The judge did not look like mercy but sounded like it. "You may stay," she said. The words struck like rain on parched earth.

I turned to her, voice trembling. "Thank you."

Outside, the city roared like it had been holding its breath. My breath was mine again. My dreams, too.

And I held them close.

Chapter 2: Familia

Securing a place in nursing school had been difficult; finding a job afterward felt Sisyphean. I passed the National Council Licensure Examination – Registered Nurse (NCLEX) a year late—my status in limbo had stalled even the taking of the exam. By then, hospitals were locking their doors tighter than vaults, and I was left knocking, invisible and unwelcome.

Before the test, a friend pressed $200 into my hand. "Pay me back when you can," he said, his belief in me a strange, fragile balm. On test day, I sat through all 265 questions. Each one blurred into the next like raindrops on a train window. I emerged into daylight blinking, unsure of my footing. I feared I had failed. I braced myself to wait more.

Days later, the results came in—I had passed. But even with a license in hand, I couldn't find a way in.

I returned to the bodega where I worked—twelve-hour shifts, seven days a week. Stocking shelves, ringing up customers, wiping the same smudges over and over. Life folded into monotony. I dreamed of fluorescents and dust.

Then Jorge Prada called. We had worked on projects together at school, his laugh always just a note louder than necessary, his optimism a kind of music. Jorge was one of the few people who never pretended—he was honest, forthcoming, and always showed up. A good friend in a time when those felt scarce.

"Come to a National Association of Hispanic Nurses (NAHN) meeting," he said.

"I'm not Hispanic."

"Doesn't matter."

So, I went.

I rode the Q train, anxiety chewing through me like moths in wool. The meeting room was alive—laughter, food, warmth. Faces turned toward me, kind and curious. I introduced myself haltingly. "Hi, I'm Zafar. I'm a nursing graduate. Jorge invited me."

A woman smiled. "We're glad you're here."

And for the first time in what felt like a century, I believed someone.

Afterward, Dan Suarez pulled me aside. "Let's meet," he said. A week later, he sat across from me in a café, nodding as I fumbled through mock interview questions. When we finished, he handed me a list of recruiters like it was a sacred text. "Follow up," he said.

He didn't have to help me. But he did.

NAHN became more than a network. It became a family. A mirror. A chorus. It taught me that giving is not a transaction—it is a promise. It reminded me that we rise by lifting others, not in theory, but in practice.

And I began to lift, too.

Chapter 3: My Calling

I wear the title nurse anesthesiologist like a quiet inheritance. It is a name I had not sought, yet one I now guard like a flame. Had you told me in nursing school this would be my future, I might've laughed, or stared blankly, trying to locate such ambition within myself.

My first glimpse of anesthesia came wrapped in sterility and awe. During an externship, I rotated through an OR where students were meant to disappear into corners. But I've never been very good at fading.

An anesthesia resident noticed me. "Who are you?" he asked. I told him.

Instead of nodding and turning away, he beckoned me beside him. A patient's blood pressure dropped; he responded without panic, explaining his steps as he worked. He placed an arterial line with the fluid grace of someone who understood not just the procedure, but its poetry. He narrated as if I were already a student of the craft. He didn't have to. But he did.

I forgot him for a while. Years passed. I worked in the ICU, grew into the rhythms of care. Then, one day, I overheard someone mention certified registered nurse anesthesiologist (CRNAs).

"What's that?"

"They're nurses. Who give anesthesia."

Oh. That's what that was.

I researched. I planned. I applied. Columbia accepted me. I arrived day one thinking the hard part was over.

How foolish. How young.

The information came like a flood. My first anesthesia pharmacology exam shattered me—67. The lowest in the class. I stopped sleeping. I made backup plans. I questioned everything.

Then I reached out to Rook, my mentor. She wrote back: "If you walk away, that's okay. But first, understand why."

Her words steadied me.

I shifted my mindset. I studied harder, yes—but more importantly, I stopped treating every exam like it was all or nothing. I reminded myself that one grade did not define me. I learned to manage fear.

On the next exam, I scored a 95.

It wasn't just the grade. It was the proof: I could stay. I could fight.

And so, I did.

Chapter 4: A Purpose That Continues

School sharpened me, but it also awakened me. In the bright rooms of academia, I saw something darker—the absence of people who looked like me, sounded like me, carried stories like mine. That silence echoed louder than lectures.

Then, in 2016, I heard Dr. Wallena Gould speak at Columbia. Her words weren't decoration; they were a call to arms. She didn't just share struggle—she spoke of transformation. She had built something: Diversity CRNA. A movement, not a moment.

After her talk, I approached her awkwardly, thanking her, unsure what I was asking for. She gave me her number. "Reach out anytime."

I did.

Later, I joined a Diversity CRNA event. I sat on a student panel, answering questions from nervous, hopeful future CRNAs. I didn't realize then how powerful presence could be. How just being there was an act of revolution.

Dr. Gould later asked if I'd join the board. I said yes, even as doubt whispered. Me?

But I did the work—reading essays, reviewing resumes, and hearing stories like echoes of my own. I realized that what we offered wasn't just guidance—it was permission.

The racism—the subtle kind, the kind that sticks like burrs—wasn't written into those essays. But I knew it lived between the lines. I had carried it.

Mentorship, I realized, wasn't kindness. It was survival. Every time I talk to a student who's unsure, nervous, second-guessing themselves—I remember that I was there once, too. They're not me, but we share threads. Sometimes all it takes is someone who remembers what it felt like to stand on the threshold.

My proudest moments come quietly. A text. An email. A phone call that starts with: "I got in." Sometimes they thank me. Sometimes they go deeper—telling me how I made them feel. That's what lasts. Not advice. Not credentials. But feeling seen.

Chapter 5: To Ammi and Papa

As I write this final chapter, I think of my parents. Of Papa, who crossed oceans so I could fly. Of Ammi, who bore pain with the silence of saints. They gave without asking. They loved without limit. Their lives were hymns of sacrifice.

I carry them in every decision. I hear them in my voice when I speak to students, in my silence when I listen. I remember Papa's heavy coat and long workdays, Ammi's soft prayers and warm hands. I remember the quiet ways they believed in me, even when I didn't believe in myself.

If there is one phrase that holds the fullness of their dream for me, it is this:

"Feet—what do I need you for when I have wings to fly? "

I have flown. Not because I was fearless, but because they believed I could. And now, I teach others to fly—not alone, not unseen—but together, toward a sky wide enough for us all.

Favorite Nursing Memory

One of my most profound memories is of a patient being transferred to the intensive care unit (ICU). As we prepared to move her, her husband turned to me, his eyes heavy with fear and hope. "Please take care of her," he said. Even now, the weight of those words lingers. In that moment, I felt the quiet, unspoken contract between a provider and a family—the trust they place in us when they have no choice but to let go. It was humbling, a reminder of the responsibility we carry, of the faith given to us when words are all they have left.

Biography

Zafar Anwar, DNP, CRNA, is an Assistant Professor at Columbia University's Doctor of Nursing Practice (DNP) in Nurse Anesthesia Program and a Certified Registered Nurse Anesthetist (CRNA) at NYPWeill Cornell Medical Center. A graduate of Columbia University's Nurse Anesthesia Program, he earned his Doctor of Nursing Practice from the University of Pennsylvania and has taught in multiple nurse anesthesia programs across the country.

With expertise in obstetric and neurosurgical anesthesia, advanced airway management, and crisis resource training, Dr. Anwar specializes in high-fidelity simulation and pharmacology education. His dedication to mentorship and representation in nurse anesthesia has led him to serve on the Board of Directors for the Diversity in Nurse Anesthesia Mentorship Program and the National Association of Hispanic Nurses – New York Chapter.

A recipient of the 2023 NAHN Forty Under 40 Leadership Award, Dr. Anwar is committed to fostering inclusivity in healthcare, mentoring future CRNAs, and advocating for equitable opportunities in the profession. Beyond clinical practice, he actively contributes to research, national presentations, and professional development initiatives. His work is driven by a deep sense of responsibility—to his patients, his students, and the next generation of diverse nurse anesthetists. He welcomes collaborations and connections via email at anwarzafar5@gmail.com.

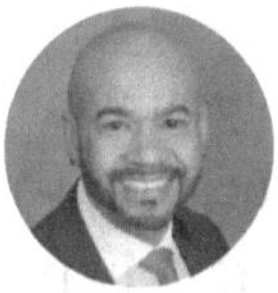

Work Hard and Enjoy Life's Rewards

JON L. MONI

"To achieve one's goals, one must have a vision, be determined, work hard, make sacrifices, and keep climbing."
– Alejandrina Collazo

Current Position

I am a Behavioral Health Home Care Nurse.

What I Love About Nursing

I love nursing because it is a profession rooted in altruism. As a nurse, I prioritize my patients' and their families' care and concerns. I enjoy advocating, educating, and empowering my patients to improve their lives. Knowing that I make a difference in my patients' lives gives me the greatest satisfaction. Nursing has also provided me with countless opportunities for personal, professional, and financial growth.

How I Got Here

I am living what I like to call an improbable life. I was born in a town called Miches, Dominican Republic, and grew up in a small rural area called Las Minas de Oro with my dad and in the city of La Romana with my mother. Growing up was difficult. I was never asked, "What do you want to be when you grow up." A future involving higher education was never in the conversation. It was me and my two sisters. My parents separated when I was a toddler, and my mother moved to La Romana with her mother. I was the youngest of the three. Around the age of 10, I remember my mother started to travel out of the country in search of a better future for her three children. Her goal was to make it to Puerto Rico, a United States (U.S.) territory, and ultimately, to the United States, and eventually bring the three of us. She knew that we would have a better future or a future period once in the U.S. She was right!

After going through many years of hardship, visas, and being deported, she finally made it to Puerto Rico, illegally. The day she was deported back to the Dominican Republic, she recalls working long hours that day as she often did and was too exhausted to get up from her bed and run from *"la migra"* as they referred to immigration agents. They caught her and sent her back. Once in Puerto Rico, she married and moved to Connecticut, United States. In 1988, she went back to the Dominican Republic to finalize her documents, which granted her legal status as a permanent resident in the United States, or her "Green Card." Her determination, hard work, and sacrifices paid off when, finally, the three of us got our "papers." We arrived in the United States in 1990 after a quick two-week stop in Puerto Rico. I remember how thrilled I was to finally be in the United States and living with my mother again.

My Journey

I was 15 years old when we arrived in the United States. I came straight to New Britain, Connecticut. Those first years were challenging, starting with the task of adjusting to the frigid winter temperatures. I missed my country, my father, my family, and my friends deeply. Not knowing the language and the culture made it more difficult to adapt. The first years of High School were challenging. I would refuse to go back to school on occasion, however, that was not an option. Mother explained to us why we must continue to attend school and assured us that things would get better. Even though neither of my parents graduated from high school, my mother believed in the power of obtaining an education. My sisters and I would go to school in the morning and return in the evening to take English as a Second Language (ESL). My mother was right, things did get better eventually.

As far as I can remember, I had great empathy for those going through hardship, especially my two sisters. As a child, I knew I wanted to have a career in the medical field. I worked at Kentucky Fried Chicken (KFC) throughout my junior and senior years in high school. Before that, I was a newspaper carrier. I did not need much English to deliver the paper, and I would have a Spanish-to English dictionary when it was time to collect the money from my clients. After high school, I went to Tunxis Community College in Farmington, CT, where I continued to take English classes and math. Because of the language barrier, I became proficient in math.

I was promoted to a full-time assistant manager position at KFC. I needed to work to help my mother, who worked two jobs. The money was good as an assistant manager, and I got to boss others around at the age of nineteen. I got married shortly after I graduated from high school. I was 21 and welcomed our son the following year. After working for a few years as an assistant manager, they offered me a position as a manager. That is when I stopped and thought about my future and my vision as a professional. Being a manager at KFC was a good opportunity with good pay, however, I knew that that was not the path I wanted to continue. My two sisters were working as Nurse Assistants then. So, I requested two weeks off from work, and I enrolled in a two-week Nurse Assistant program. When I got my Nurse Assistant Certificate, I saw that as the first step in healthcare. I worked in different nursing homes and enjoyed caring for the elderly. I also worked as a Home Health Aide for a short period. By now, it was clear to me what I wanted to be "when I grew up." I wanted to be a nurse.

Let The Journey Begin

I enrolled in a Licensed Practical Nurse program (LPN) in 1999. The LPN program I applied for was full-time, Monday to Friday in the morning, and clinical some evenings. It was not easy as I had to support my family. Thanks to the support of my in-laws at that time, I completed the program in the year 2000. I received the Director's Award from the faculty. I was happy to graduate. I began working as a visiting nurse in the community and longterm care facilities after earning my LPN license, I kept climbing. Five years later, I enrolled in a bridge program LPN to registered nurse (RN) at Excelsior College, now known as Excelsior University. In 2007, I graduated with my Associate Nursing Degree (ASN). The bridge program was great. You get to control the pace at which you complete the program. I put in a lot of effort and time, and I was able to complete the program in 2 years. It was a proud moment. When I got my registered nurse license, I took time to reflect on how lucky I was to have chosen nursing as my profession. I continue to work in home care as a medical-surgical nurse. As a medical-surgical home care nurse, I provide skilled nursing care to patients recovering from surgery, managing chronic illnesses, or dealing with acute medical conditions in their homes. I also educate patients and their families on chronic disease prevention and management, medication adherence, and lifestyle modifications. Additionally, I worked in collaboration with their providers, physical therapists, and other healthcare professionals to develop a comprehensive, patient-centered care plan that provided compassionate support, promoted recovery, prevented hospital readmissions, and helped patients regain their independence and return to their normal lives. Some patients require acute care, and some have chronic conditions and require long-term care. Home care nurses play a crucial role in improving patient outcomes and reducing healthcare costs by providing continuous monitoring and intervention.

As a home health nurse, I am involved in the community and collaborate with different organizations in the community, providing my patients and their families with resources to help improve their lives. There is a need for behavioral health male nurses in the community. I've seen the need, and for the past 12 years, I have been working as a psychiatric home care nurse. I work with a very diverse population, most of whom have chronic mental disorders like depression, bipolar, post-traumatic stress disorder (PTSD), schizophrenia, schizo-affective, substance abuse, etc. As a behavioral health home care nurse, I provide specialized care to individuals managing psychiatric disorders in their home environment. I assess my patients' mental and emotional well-being, monitor medication adherence, provide crisis intervention, and offer therapeutic support to help manage and improve symptoms. It is gratifying when your patients' quality of life improves; they are empowered to manage their conditions, reduce stigma, and gain stability and independence.

Latino home care nurses have a significant impact on their patients, their families, and the community by providing culturally competent, compassionate care that meets the unique needs of Latino patients. As a bilingual advocate, we help bridge language and cultural gaps, ensuring better communication, trust, and health outcomes, reducing healthcare disparities, and improving access to essential services. By addressing cultural stigmas around mental health and medical care, we encourage more individuals to seek treatment. Latino nurses' presence fosters representation, empowerment, and stronger community connections, making healthcare more inclusive and accessible for all.

On July 12, 2024, I climbed another step. I graduated from Excelsior University in Albany, New York, with a Bachelor of Science in Nursing (BSN). It was a long journey, and I had to go through a lot of obstacles, but I did it because I had a vision, was determined, worked hard, and made sacrifices. I am grateful for the support my family and close friends provided. I always tell anyone who is considering pursuing a profession in nursing but is unsure to go ahead and start. Ask for support from your loved ones and the school. Don't be discouraged; don't let difficulties and barriers stop you from achieving your objective. The nursing profession provides unlimited opportunities for personal and professional growth. Nursing has also helped me achieve financial freedom and provide for my family.

Several years ago, the state of Connecticut proposed to reduce or eliminate funds to a community-based program that provided daily medication administration to behavioral health patients who would otherwise not take their medication, putting them at high risk for self-harm and hospitalization. On several occasions, I participated in going to the Legislative Building in Hartford, CT, with a group of community nurses and nurse leaders to lobby lawmakers to keep the program funded. Some changes were made; however, mental health patients continue to benefit from this program today. One of my aspirations for my future in nursing is to be influential and advocate for my patients at the legislative level.

My Favorite Nursing Memory

As a visiting nurse, I have made a difference in my patients' and their families' lives by providing direct care in an intimate setting. I get to build meaningful relationships by providing individualized care and support. Unlike hospital settings with shorter patient interactions, I build a strong therapeutic relationship with my patients and their families. I have great memories of being there for my patient and their family for a significant number of years, going to funerals, birthdays, weddings, and celebrating anniversaries. Some of my patients have embraced me as another family member.

Biography

Jon L. Moni, BSN, RN, was born and raised in the Dominican Republic. Jon migrated to the United States in 1990 alongside his two older sisters, driven by his mother's unwavering vision, determination, and sacrifices. Settling in New Britain, CT, he has seized the opportunities this country offers, for which he's grateful, working diligently toward his goals. Today, he resides in West Hartford, CT. He is the proud dad to his son, Johan L. Moni.

Jon's journey in nursing began in 2000 when he earned his Licensed Practical Nurse (LPN) license from Lincoln Technical Institute. His passion for healthcare led him to pursue further education, earning an Associate of Science in Nursing (ASN) in 2007. In 2023, he achieved a significant milestone, earning his Bachelor of Science in Nursing (BSN) from Excelsior University. He's committed to lifelong learning.

Jon is passionate about nursing. He is committed to making a meaningful impact on the lives of his patients, ensuring they receive the care, guidance, and advocacy needed to thrive in their homes and the community. A proud Latino, Jon values the unique perspective and cultural richness he brings to the nursing profession. He is grateful for the unwavering support of his family and close friends.

In his free time, Jon enjoys spending quality time with his family and friends. He enjoys traveling. However, his favorite destination remains the Dominican Republic, where he reconnects with family. Whether discovering new cultures or simply enjoying the company of loved ones, Jon finds joy in creating meaningful experiences wherever he goes. He welcomes collaborations and connections via email at jonmoni@gmail.com.

PS Gracias, Madre!

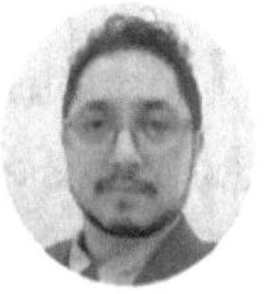

Resiliency

THOMAS MARQUES

"If it was easy, it wouldn't be fun!"

Current Position

I am an Emergency Department (ED) Nurse.

What I love About Nursing

No two days are the same. Some are good, some are bad, but in the end, I know I did my best to help people, and that's what I love most about all of this.

Myself

How did I become a nurse? It is the question I have been asking myself for the past years, especially thinking on my background as an engineer.

My name is Thomas Marques, an upper 30s male naturalized from Brazil, who always had a taste for adventures, outside activities, spending time with people and animals, and automotive stuff. My very first dream was to become a sport car driver, but it was quite difficult to achieve, so I decided to become an engineer. I must assume that since my young age, I was always with minor injuries and scratches after my "not-too-careful adventures and playtime." I always enjoyed giving my friends and myself first aide, as I liked to see everybody feeling better, healing, and getting ready for the next "trouble time." For my transition from middle to high school, I had the option to apply for a technical nursing school, something similar to a Licensed Practical Nurse program; however, nursing is a career that unfortunately is not really well recognized and paid in Brazil. At 15 years old, I was looking for a way to achieve financial independency. Even though biology was something that fascinated me, the fact of having to memorize a lot of information was something that scared me. To make it short, I became a Mechatronics Technologist and later a Mechanical Engineer in 2011.

The Turning Point

Things were going well, and I was really enjoying my career; however, a great crisis in my country put myself and many others in layoffs. With a reduced market and a great difficulty returning to the automotive industry at that time, I decided to get in contact with some cousins who have been living in Connecticut. They readily offered me support to move and engage with college to improve my English skills. In 2017, I began my English as a Second Language (ESL) classes. That same year, I injured my leg resulting in an infection. We all know how difficult it is to access health support in the US, but luckily a friend referred me to a free community free clinic in Danbury. After being helped, I offered to volunteer to the clinic, which put me in contact with patients and the community on a weekly basis.

Time passed by and I was about to graduate from the local Community College with my ESL certificate. The original plan was to return to Brazil and use my language knowledge, as I also learned Spanish from the contact with native speakers and to return to the automotive industry However, supporting people became a great part of myself. At this point, the clinic staff, including the director, were encouraging me to pursue a nursing career, as they could see a great nurse in me. My college advisors were also telling me the same, as my learning capacity, critical thinking, and people and procedure skills could be well applicable. I was not confident enough until a specific event. A friend had a baby, but her C-section got infected, and she needed to spend a week at the hospital. She did not speak a single word of English at that time, and her family could not stay with her all the time as they need to take care of the baby, who was home. I offered to stay overnight with her, and this gave me the taste of a nursing career. I had contact with numerous procedures like medication administration, blood transfusion, wound care, and others. I also had great chats with nurses, assistants, and even doctors.

Nursing School

Even with my fear of biology terminology and memorization, I decided to register for General Studies for pre-nursing requirements. Pursuing a major in a second language means learning not just the subject, but the vocabulary related to it, which requires more effort. My engineering background gave me great logical thinking, causes and consequences strategies, and problem solve mechanisms, which helped me a lot with biology subject matter. Once the time came, I was ready to apply for one of the most competitive nursing programs, passing on my first attempt. In a class with 120 people, even with other immigrants, I was the only student who the English knowledge was about 5 years old, and one of the few who never actually worked in the medical field.

Nursing school was not easy. It was the hardest academic period of my life so far, with a great amount of intellectual and practical content in a short period of time, extensive lectures, deep subjects, hard exams, hands-on clinicals dealing with patients and staff, and no space for mistakes. Instructors push us as hard as they can to extract the best of us, but unfortunately not all of them think in the same way, at least until you prove yourself. More than once, I needed to deal with people who did not see or could not accept me as a nurse, including some instructors. Semester by semester, I proved myself and improved my knowledge and skills, earning good grades without any failure, eventually nominated to be the school senate representative for the 2023 National Student Nurse Association (NSNA) convention, representing not only my college but the state of Connecticut at the annual seminar. But again, not everybody seems to agree with our success.

During my last semester, I faced the first person who made me feel incapable of becoming a nurse. A longtime career as a nurse and an educator, someone with incredible knowledge and great lecture skills, but with a debatable sense of equity. My knowledge, skills, personality, gender, and accent did not seem sufficient or suitable for her. In a group of 8 clinical students, being the only male and heavy accent speaker, I was always the one in trouble, who the skills were not good enough, the reports were not accepted, the communication were not understandable, the one she always had something to complain about, the only one who was never allowed to clinical rotations to get familiar with other sections of the hospital such ICU and ED, despite all the 7 girls have done it twice, among many other situations. Even the nurses in the clinical setting asked me what I had done, because the instructor was clearly picking on me.

She was my first breaking point. Even other immigrant students shared with me similar situations with the same instructor, but they all were scared to do something. These situations were consuming me, affecting my concentration, my grades, and my dedication to the NCLEX. At that point, I was already hired by the same hospital I was doing my clinicals, because according to the HR, the coordinators and charge nurses had already liked my performance during clinicals and even the Chief Nursing Officer (CNO) knew me by name. How could the hospital consider me a good nurse and my instructor threatened me with failure at the same time? Something was wrong and I could not let this interrupt my dream.

I have not officially reported the instructor, but I have had good conversations with some other school staff that I trust. In summary, they all encouraged me to talk to her in person, just us, as they all trust my soft skills for advocacy with respect. And I did so! One day, after clinic, I asked for a private conversation. I made my point as respectful as possible, listed some examples, explained how it all was affecting me, and how my experience contradicted my grades and achievements prior to our interaction. Of course, she denied everything, but was surprised and glad that I preferred to talk to her before submitting a report, as other students did in the past (yes, she already had several reports for similar reasons). It was all before spring break, and when we came back for the last half of the semester, everything was different! She continued to be a demanding instructor, but in a healthy and completely different way than before. She actually became really supportive, almost with a proud aura. One day, when I was working at the ED, I passed by her and her new group of students and told them how happy and excited I was with my new role as a night shift ED nurse, and how much she prepared me for the real life, and with a good smile, she said how proud she was. I earned her respect.

Registered Nurse

My graduation was certainly one of the happiest days of my life. It is really weird and difficult to explain to your family and friends how happy you are but still stressed and not able to fully celebrate your achievement prior to taking the licensing exam. You are not a nurse until you earn the right to use a "RN" after your name. And to make this moment even more special, the National Council Licensure ExaminationRN (NCLEX) decided to change the exam model in the Summer 2023, the year I was applying for my license. What could be more satisfying than to take a brand new test, with several changes that no one has seen in real practice, and even some of the people who were supposed to understand the test model had doubts about how things will really work in practice? Adrenaline was in great demand at this time. Yes, I did pass! Come on, I did not get here to leave a national exam, with a high level of specific knowledge, highly protected, full of "never seen before" scenarios, timed to prevent me from getting my dream license. I could finally celebrate…but not for too long.

As I mentioned before, I was hired for a night shift position at the ED of the same hospital I did my clinicals. A position that is not easily offered to new graduates as it requires special training and fast learning pace, which usually comes after some years of experience in settings like Medical-Surgical units. However, my hiring process was unusual, because as a visa holder, my Temporary Work Visa at that time allowed me to work for 12 months only, and then, must be replaced with a long-term working visa, which requires a legal and financial sponsor. I started to work in August 2023, the most exciting occupation I ever had. Every day there was something new! From handing Acetaminophen to people with headaches that decided to go to ED at 3am before taking a pill at home, to multiple car accidents bringing more than 1 person in with full trauma alerts. Bringing people back to life after cardiac arrests, seeing Emergency Medical Technicians (EMTs) running with woman in active delivery to the maternity floor, helping doctors apply pressure to femoral arteries until the proper device was placed, holding babies and little kids to place an intravenous (IV) access, seeing sick kids smiling after a silly joke, dodging punches from the elderly when we are just trying to clean them up, bring tea to the same elderly person that now wants to tell you about their grandkids, seeing naked patients running around, helping families to see their loved one, and many other cases with happy and bad ends (most of them happy) helped me to solidify my previous thoughts, to make sure this is my calling and what I want to do for a great part of my life: be a nurse and help people!

Working Visa?

However, my nursing journey has been full of barriers, and here is the latest one: My long-term working visa is pending in the immigration office. All the paperwork and bureaucracy has been done and submitted in proper time, but now, it all depends on the immigration department. Members from the hospital, college, and even Senators have tried to help me, but there is nothing else to be done besides waiting, for an average time between 1-3 years. It is March 2025 and so far, it has been 6 months since I've had to stop working and about 7 months that my process has no updates. I still have my passion, and I miss the hospital every day, but I know it is just another breaking point, and like the other ones, I will overcome this too and return to work as a nurse, whether here or in another country that gives me the opportunity. After all, not all places apply barriers for nurses.

Favorite Nursing Memory

I am a big fan of Anime and I keep a figure of my favorite character on my badge holder. One night I was assigned a family concerned about their 5-year-old son who was experiencing testicular pain. We needed to examine, but the boy was afraid. The Father saw my badge and we started to talk about Anime. The boy relaxed and showed me his underwear with the same Anime. With no hesitation, I said "Nice, you have a dragon taking care of your balls!" His mother and the doctor lost it. The father and kid were laughing and crying, and he finally let us examine him!

Biography

Naturalized from Brazil, Thomas Marques, RN is a 38 year-old male who needed to become an engineer to understand that he has always been a nurse. After living 30 years in his mother country where he earned a Bachelor of Mechanical Engineering and a Master of Project Management, Thomas decided to go abroad to learn and experience new languages and cultures and ended learning much more about himself. During his 6 years at the Community College, he was a dedicated student worker and a mentor, especially for students with Latino heritage. He also played important roles at Latinos and Nursing clubs, including being the national representation at the 2023 National Student Nurse Association (NSNA) convention. Being part of the great Danbury community, Thomas was a longtime volunteer at a local free healthcare clinic, where he was encouraged to pursuit his nursing career. He offered great support to the local community during the COVID-19 pandemic and is also known as a frequent blood and platelets donor. He believes in a better society when people help each other with the best of they can. He is someone who likes challenges that can result in personal growth. He has a cat named Kion and enjoys some adrenaline with motorsport activities and outdoor adventures. He welcomes collaborations and connections via email at marquesthomas1986@gmail.com and on social at linkedin.com/in/thomasmarquesrnmbab75848a6 and @marquesthomas1986.

About The Author

Dr. Tina Loarte-Rodríguez (she|her|ella) is a nurse, educator, author, advocate, and visionary whose life and work are rooted in purpose: *leave the world better than you found it.* With over 19 years of experience in clinical practice and leadership, she is a transformative force in healthcare—boldly leading with compassion, equity, and unshakable resolve.

Born into a working-class family, Tina was raised in a home where money was tight, but dreams were expansive. Her parents taught her that kindness, education, and faith in something bigger could carry you through anything. That foundation lit a fire in her—a tenacity for more, for better, for justice.

She pursued that calling through education, earning degrees from Cornell University, the University of Connecticut, and Quinnipiac University. Her academic path reflects her blend of rigorous scholarship and relentless advocacy, and her work is a living testimony to what happens when intellect and heart work in harmony.

Tina is proud of her identity as an Afro-Latina Boricua, and she brings her whole, authentic self to everything she does. She is evolving at the various intersections of being Human, embracing her many roles as author, advocate, Belonging and Health Equity practitioner, eternal learner, and optimist. Her leadership is powered by kindness, driven by innovation, rooted in wellness, and sustained by self-care.

As the creator of the *Latinos in Nursing* anthology series, she is reclaiming space, amplifying silenced stories, and honoring the brilliance of Latino nurses—especially those who have been historically excluded from the narrative. Through her work, she is not just telling stories; she is building a movement.

A proud mother and a revolution in motion, Dr. Loarte Rodríguez shows us what it looks like to lead with heart, to fight with purpose, and to rise with community. Her work is not only a gift to the profession—it is a gift to the world.

This book is her offering. Her legacy. And just the beginning.

She welcomes collaborations and connections via email at tina@latinasinnursing.org.

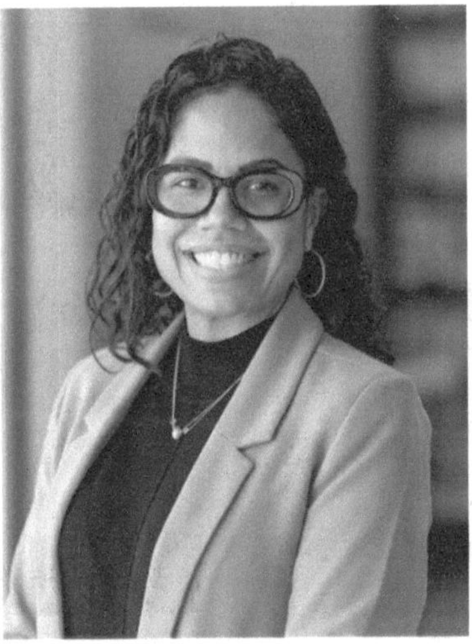

Dra. Tina Loarte-Rodríguez

Latinos in Nursing Contributing Authors

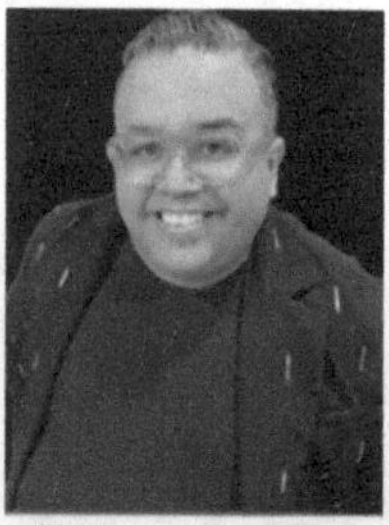
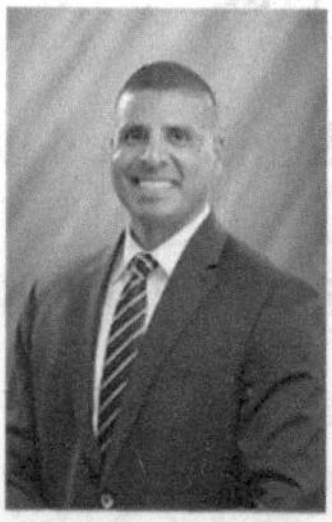
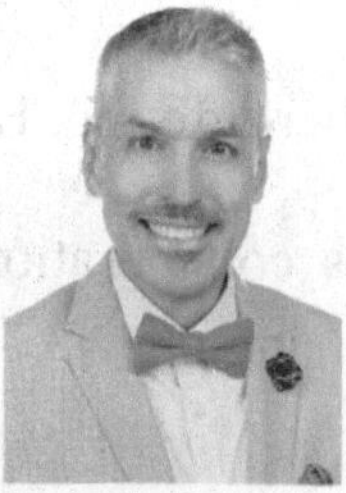
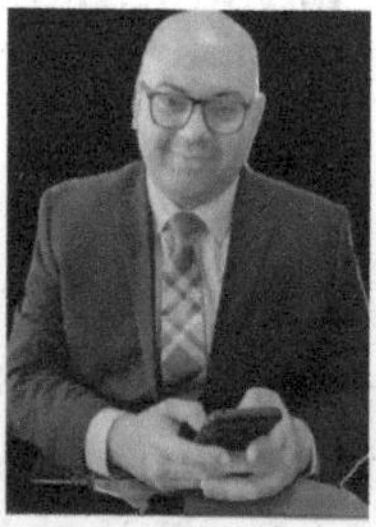
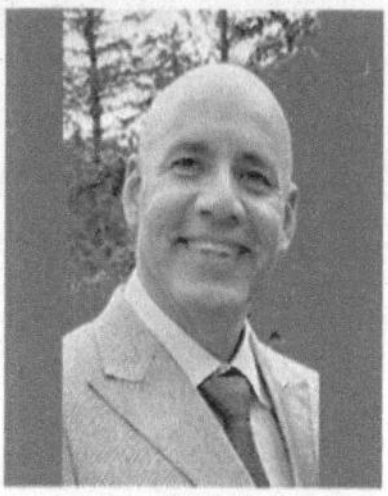
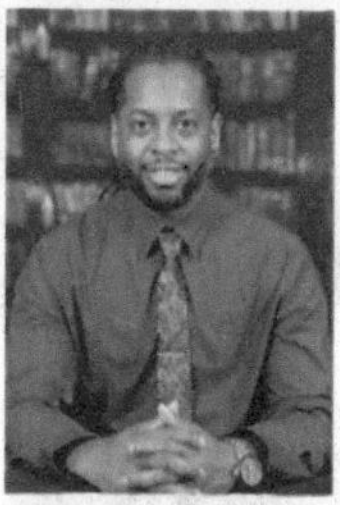
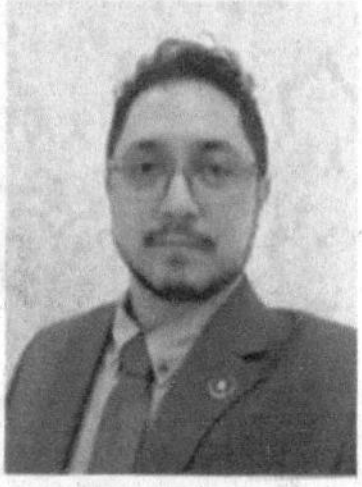
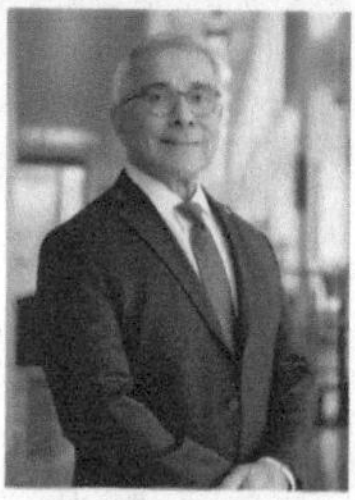
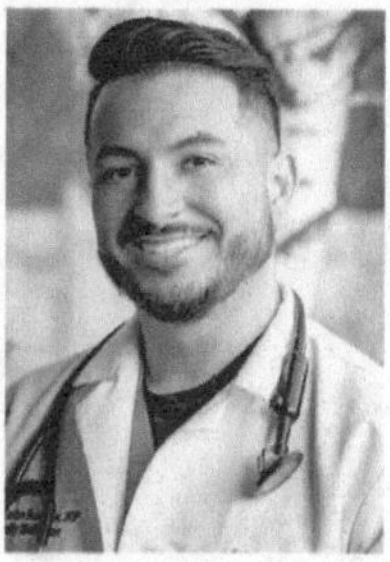
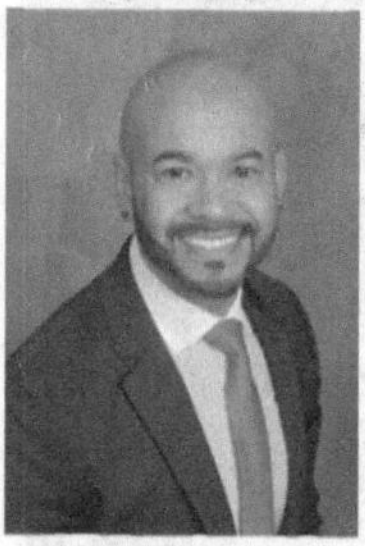
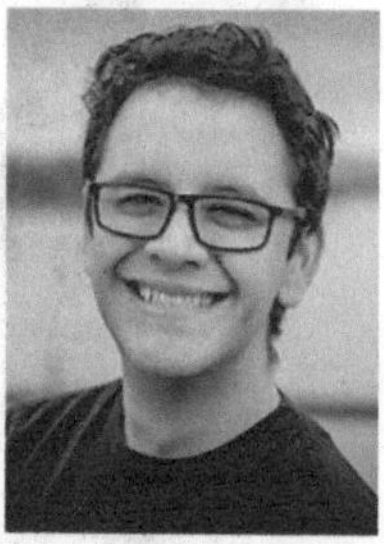
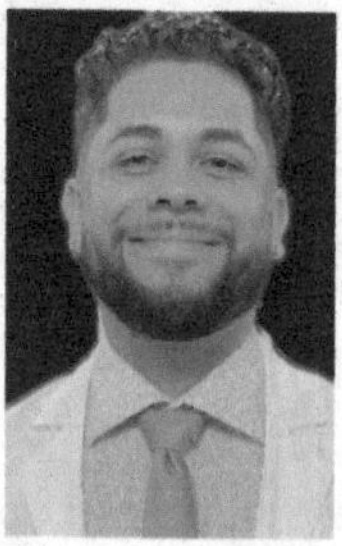